BLUE-COLLAR BEAUTY

Confessions of a Plastic Surgery Coach

Michelle Emmick

memmick@mycoachmd.com

The stories contained in this book are true. I recreated events, locales and conversations from my memories of them. In order to maintain their anonymity, I have changed the names of individuals, places and identifying characteristics and details such as physical properties, occupations and places of residence.

Book Design and Edits

by Michelle Morrow

www.chellreads.com

1st round edits: Lianne Laroque

Paperback ISBN: 978-1-7341343-0-8

EBook ISBN: 978-1-7341343-1-5

Dedication

To my bright, smart, kind, funny, cool, determined, adventurous, compassionate, entertaining, tenacious, talkative, unique, logical, sensitive, positive, gifted, beautiful and loved Daughter, Carson Win.

Table of Contents

Author's Note

I have worked in the aesthetic industry close to 20 years, performed over 10,000 consultations, trained over 2000 practice team members, and have personally generated over 30 million dollars in sales. I've held leadership positions for many of the large retail medical brands, private practice plastic surgeons, and medical spas. Over the last two years, I've transitioned to building my own company working with people throughout the US and internationally. My passion has always been two-fold; support consumers on their aesthetic journey and provide business the right coaching to drive results. I have seen a lot of so-called experts in this industry. People who offer trainings, speaking engagements and have high profile social media. I believe everyone is a subject matter expert in something. Mine happens to be in the aesthetic space when it comes to understanding how to have or provide a great patient experience. I feel fortunate to transfer my knowledge to empower others as their coach.

I worked for the largest national plastic surgery chain. We were the first aesthetics company to leverage marketing and were known as the industry disruptors and pioneers to what would ultimately become a game-changer for the aesthetics industry. This is my experience of the rise and fall of Lifestyle Lift and all the years between and after. It's a book about my personal story and journey as a Plastic Surgery Coach, which I would consider a bit of a memoir. It was written as my love letter to a profession and the people that mean so much to me. A career that has brought me an opportunity to connect with so many people. People with unique stories, no two the same. I have changed names and identifying details of the characters portrayed in the book however all the stories are 100% true.

I couldn't have done it without her. The loyalty and enthusiasm she brought inside the company and to the patients was invaluable. Michelle shaped the culture of Lifestyle Lift to one of the greatest ones in the country. I have a deep respect for her and the value she continues to bring to the medical aesthetic industry.

-Dr. David Kent

Prologue

"Really, mom, you couldn't buy me a bigger size?"

"What? It was cute?"

"Nothing cute about my belly hanging over my ready to pop Garanimals® shorts."

"Well, what was I gonna do? You wore your sisters hand me downs. Plus, you always loved to eat! We couldn't keep snacks in the house."

A little chubster—yep, that was me. As a kid, I lived for when mom came home with those perfectly wrapped silver Ding Dongs®. My favorite thing to do as a little girl was to lay down on the brown shag carpet, and watch TV shows. You could always find me with a giant bowl of Corn Flakes®—Lucky Charms® if it was payday. Don't get me wrong—I was an active child. I played piano, softball,

Brownies/Girl Scouts—everything a normal little kid liked to do But, staring at a box that transported me to different worlds and different people while enjoying my favorite treats, now that was happiness.

Fast-forward to high school. I finally slimmed down after joining the swim team. My love for food hadn't changed, but I was burning calories, and I got lean. I held my weight until the college freshman 15 crept up. My favorite story was when my friends and I planned a spring break trip. We drove from Buffalo, NY to Panama City, Florida. Since we were going to have to wear bathing suits, we started our SlimFast™ diet 3 weeks before (because that's plenty of time to lose weight). What's sad is we weren't what you would consider fat, however, as most college-aged girls, we thought we were. We stayed strict with our diet drinking our 3 shakes a day. I can't imagine we restrained from drinking though that would have been a big stretch. We hit the tanning booth a few times, and with our new slender selves, we were feeling good. We packed up the car to start a ridiculously long road trip. We didn't make it out of the state of NY before we were in line at Wendy's drive-thru.

That story was twenty-five years ago, and I would say I consider myself a professional dieter. I say diet, the dirty word. I'm supposed to say a lifestyle change—healthy eating. I know, and I do those things. I work out regularly and diet too. I wish I could say I didn't gain and lose the same 20lbs since college, but that would be a lie. When I was pregnant with my daughter, I gained a ridiculous amount of weight. Since I was older, I fell into the high-risk pregnancy category. Being the emotional eater that I tend to be, and the constant worrying if the baby was okay, I became intimate with late night mint chocolate chip ice cream. It started to become a nightly ritual for me. Open the freezer, grab a spoon, pop off the top and go all in. We all know you're not supposed to eat late at night or in front of the television, but there I was reverting back to those days as a little girl. I didn't know if I would ever get back to a place where I liked myself. I called my friend Jenny... you may know her Jenny Craig, and off I went. Close to 100lbs later and a lot of hard work, I got myself back. Eight years later, I've lost another 100...gaining and losing year after year that same 20 lbs. The struggle is real.

I tell this story because while it's not plastic surgery, it relates so well. It's that connection I feel to others when they come to me not feeling their best. Those people who have a story, whether from being a young girl or a grown woman. That feeling of 'I want to make a positive change, for me.'

This is where I identified. This is where I made the connection, and found my calling as a young woman starting in the aesthetic industry. It's part of my story.

Chapter 1: Defining Beauty

When did everyone start looking alike? Between the make-up contouring, lighting, and, filters we're becoming a land of dolls. When did individuality get lost? Are we so enamored with outside influences and ridiculous standards of distorted beauty that we're losing the true essence of what makes us unique?

Merriam-Webster's Dictionary Definition of **Beauty**: "*The quality or aggregate of qualities in a person or thing that gives pleasure to the senses or pleasurably exalts the mind or spirit: loveliness.*"[1]

Who and what define beauty? When it comes to appearance, there are different perceptions of what is considered beautiful. However, the more and more we turn to the Internet and social media, our standard of beauty starts to blend.

---

1 https://www.merriam-webster.com/dictionary/beauty

We have a select group of people setting the standard, and people are following like soldiers. We buy magazines that claim the world's most beautiful people. Why are they considered beautiful? Because they have a great plastic surgeon and a cosmetic dentist? We've got plus size clothing. Why? Because not everyone is a size 2. We don't all have bodies like supermodels. So, why, when it comes to plastic surgery, every website or Instagram post or Facebook advertisement is showing a woman with perfect skin, no cellulite, washboard abs, in a string bikini? Who is this person? Nobody I'm walking by at the grocery store or standing in line at the deli counter. I haven't seen her in the Chic-Fil-A drive-thru. She's not at my daughter's school PTA meeting. We can't relate to these images, yet they keep shoving them in our faces. When is it enough, and when do we say, "let's make some adjustments?" I'm not asking for an extreme change, just something more realistic to what is real-world.

What about the everyday beauty? The get up every day, go to my job, take kids to practice, and throw a load of laundry that's been sitting in the basket all week into the wash, make a box of macaroni and cheese for dinner beauty? Where is she?

The plastic surgery industry, and all aesthetics, for that matter, sell us the ideal. Beauty comes in all shapes and sizes and should be celebrated and properly represented. I represent what the business and political world call the blue-collar folks. Yes, that's right. The unpretentious, everyday people that want to look and feel their best.

I've spent almost 20 years in the field of aesthetic beauty. I've met with over 10,000 men and women, old, young, rich, and poor. I've socialized with the rich and famous, and I've consulted with women who don't have a dime in their pocket. I've watched how the definition of beauty has changed and how it's easy to be influenced by what we're being force-fed.

Here's what I've learned about beauty. We are all unique and beautiful. If you want surgery, have surgery. If you want to make a change or enhance your looks, do it. I don't care if it's coloring your hair, piercing your ears, or getting bigger boobs—do what makes you happy. What you need to be certain of is that happiness comes from within—from your life experience and the people you share those experiences with. The things that you are excited and passionate about. What evokes feelings of love and goodness.

I think Webster's dictionary got it right. Now read it again.

CHAPTER 2: My Story

"You're so nice and normal looking. I mean, don't get me wrong—you're very pretty; it's just I was expecting someone... you know... that looks like they've had a lot of plastic surgery." This always makes me laugh; I get it, and thank you. I represent the other side. The everyday I go to Target or Walmart to pick up my kids' school supplies kind of plastic surgery coach. At any given time, I could have a stain on my shirt from a toddler's sticky fingers. I'm a 46-year-old college-educated, wife, and mom. I clean up well but look like a homeless person without my hair and makeup done plastic surgery consultant. Yep, that's me.

I'm also a coach. A great one. God's given me the authentic ability to connect with people, and I've taken my skills to start my own business MyCoachMD. Being able to choose the best people to work with and the people I know have a genuine heart and passion for the aesthetic industry, has been priceless. The people who want to help others look and feel their best; who want to educate them on the procedures and services out there, and if anything, point them in the right direction. And if they need us, allow us to coach them every step of the way.

CHAPTER 3: The Fall

Wall Street Journal, March 2015: Lifestyle Lift, a nationwide chain of cosmetic surgery centers, abruptly shut down the majority of its business Monday and said it is considering filing for bankruptcy.

The company, founded in 2001 by Dr. David Kent, had 40 surgery centers nationwide offering what it billed as a less-invasive face-lift procedure that required only local anesthesia and shorter recovery times. Its advertisements boasted that the services are affordable for everyday people who want to "look as young on the outside as you feel on the inside."

My heart was broken. If you've ever been a part of something you loved so much, worked tirelessly for and believed so strongly in, then watch it end, is like going through a divorce, break up, or whatever that pit in your stomach turn-the-knife churning I want to burst into tears feeling is. I'd been gone four years, and that was still how it felt.

I was 29 years old when I started working at Lifestyle Lift. I took a job as a Patient Consultant. After a few short months of working with four different plastic surgeons, I moved my way up the corporate ladder to Head of Sales. I spent the next 5 1/2 years flying all over the United States opening new locations, hiring, coaching, and training more people than I can remember. I was full of the 'I can do anything mentality,' and I said yes to everything. Every process and procedure to develop, job description, training material, committee, every new idea to implement, there I was! Bright-eyed, determined, ready to sink my teeth in. My nickname was the Golden Child.

Looking back, why wouldn't I have been? I worked like a circus animal and made everyone around me look less than. Thankfully, I was well-liked and respected, or else I probably would have been hated. I know I would have given someone like me the stink eye. "Calm down girl—it's not a race." Now that I'm older and a parent, I have a much more 'work smarter, not harder' work life balance mentality. Back then, I had no idea and truly believed it was one of the reasons the company was as successful as it was. We had high expectations, and everyone on our leadership team stepped up to the challenge. The 'let me prove I'm a winner' mentality never slowed down. I was flying from city to city, making more money than both my schoolteacher parents combined.

What's funny is that these days, I barely hop on a plane unless I have too. I check for a direct flight and turn down offers based on whether it works within my lifestyle. Back then, it was easy to run on autopilot. I used to have two suitcases. Come home on Friday, drop my bag and pick up the next one for Monday morning onto the next state. It was hard work, but it was exhilarating. The company had a sense of family, and we built something like no one had done before.

Our founder was a visionary and pioneer who took a lot of ridicule in those early days inside the medical community. How could someone market a medical procedure? An infomercial? Blasphemy! Industry insiders dismissed us. To them, we had zero credibility. We were outcasts and the "Pony Boy" outsiders to a world of elitists. But to those of us from the inside, a company based in Michigan, with people like me from Elmira, a small town in Upstate New York where plastic surgery is not common; we knew we were building something special.

We traveled the country meeting with hardworking, everyday Americans who wanted to look and feel their best. We knew we could offer them a lot more than looking years younger. We were changing lives. I remember attending a society meeting one year in California, looking to recruit more doctors for our new practices. There we stood like Pigpen in a Charlie Brown movie. They didn't want to give us an exhibitor booth. It was like our money was dirty and we weren't allowed inside the country club. We knew who we were, and we didn't care. We took it in stride when we realized that we had been given a spot practically in the hallway. Oh well, we set up our well-hidden booth with a "nobody puts baby in the corner mentality" and rocked it. What was funny about that story is how many doctors secretly contacted us. They didn't want their colleagues to know they were interested. But let's face it, we had been dominating the market, and everybody was interested.

I had a true love affair with that business and its people. And just like any relationship, over time, things changed. To me, it became different. There became new dynamics that entered the family, and most of us tried hard to cling to what we once had, but it was drifting. I didn't like the direction. It was like watching your best friend dating a bad boy, and no matter how much you pleaded for her to stay away, she wouldn't listen.

Now, you can't blame one person in a relationship—there are always flaws on both sides. However, when you pull away from the people who keep you safe and guide you, things are gonna happen. Being fiercely loyal and a fixer by nature, I tried dealing with it and even changed my role inside the organization. I contemplated leaving and would play it over and over. How can I leave my family? Everything we've built. That voice in my head and that feeling in my gut said, "Michelle, it's time." I was becoming resentful, and that wasn't who I was or wanted to be. And just like a person stays in a relationship too long, I understood deep down it was time to turn off the sad love song and let go. Eventually, I made the hardest career decision to date. I said goodbye.

I learned so much from my days at Lifestyle Lift. A place that provided me amazing opportunities and relationships that have paved my way through the course of my professional career. I have worked for quite a few different companies over the years. The common thread for me has always been the people and the stories along the way—both colleagues and patients. The stories that make you laugh and cry. The emotionally uplifting and the heartbreaking stories are beyond special to me because it grows you as a person. I've experienced the good, bad, and ugly of plastic surgery.

CHAPTER 4: Lose Yourself

Before my start in plastic surgery, I spent several years working in the weight loss industry. I always reference this as where I built my foundation and my deep connection with people. I started as a sales counselor and moved into management and training quickly. If you don't know, the US weight loss market is an over 60-billion-dollar industry. That's three times the market on plastic surgery. Back in the 90s and early 2000s, weight loss companies popped up everywhere. Now, many people use online apps or participate in multi-level marketing programs. But back then, if you were overweight, you signed up for a program that promoted losing 2-3 lbs. a week, and you were instructed to follow a strict program, weigh in weekly, and meet with your counselor. I started my career as a Counselor. I didn't have a background in counseling; however, I did get my undergraduate degree in social work, and boy was I using my skills. Day in and day out, I would listen to people's struggles, reading their food diary entries.

"Really Jen, you ate an entire bag of Cheetos and a frozen pizza? Girl, I feel you. I love me some frozen pizza!"

I mean, come on, sometimes you just had to cut them some slack. I got it because I've struggled with my weight my entire life. I love food. It's the biggest drug out there, and here I was, 26-year-old counseling others on how to stop their drug habit when I couldn't stop the bad habits myself. Cabbage soup, grapefruit diet, that nasty lemonade maple syrup diets, please, I've done them all!

I used to tell my clients I was going to open a clothing store called 2 to 12 because that covered all the sizes I could wear in a given year. The clients loved me because I understood them. I did the program right along with them and shared their successes and setbacks. The goal was always to get back up and keep going, and I always pushed them forward with empathy and encouragement. This was coaching at its finest, but I didn't know that at the time. I just did what came naturally. I often found some of the clients came in just to have someone to talk to. I can tell you there is nothing any therapist has on me, and quite frankly, I could receive an honorary degree from Harvard University with my listening skills. From my time in weight loss, we had some great success stories. We sold products to try to overcome any craving and pills to block the fat.

I moved up quickly to training and management because I was good. But for me, it just felt easy and second nature. Back then; the company provided training on how to overcome objections and how to present price packages to clients. Every statement came with a response, and they asked us to memorize it. It seemed silly to me, but the words made sense. I mean, if someone says that package is too much money, I would respond, "Naturally," with, "I understand how you feel. It is a big investment. Aren't you here for the big investment? Why would you sign up for a package that's only getting you halfway to goal? If you're going to commit, let's do this, go all in, right?" The higher-ups loved me. They used to put baby monitors in the rooms to listen to our conversations. We didn't have sophisticated technology back then; we didn't even have computers in our offices.

I remember my boss coming in after my conversation with the client. She was extremely animated and fun. She had lost a ton of weight and wore her hair super short and wore bright colors. She would come into my office with her arms stretched out slow clapping, "Well done, Michelle. You are such a superstar. "Thanks." I need you to teach everyone else how to do and say what you do to get people excited about making a positive change for themselves.

The program worked for some and not so much for others. We had clients who would sign up year after year, struggling to lose the same weight or rejoining because they gained some or all of their weight back. I felt for them and related because of my yo-yo dieting. I'm like a bear that gets ready to hibernate for the winter. Look pretty good in the summer, then October rolls around—forget it. I basically turn into a pumpkin. If it has pumpkin in it, I'm in. Pumpkin muffins, pumpkin cookies, pumpkin pie, and I recently heard they are making Pumpkin pie Halo top ice cream! Dear Jesus, take the wheel!

I was listening to people's same struggles as mine and really wanted to encourage and help. It was a job, and we worked long hours, typically six days a week, but it was a job I cared about and enjoyed. I knew that with each client, we had to get to the heart of the issues—the source of emotion causing the bad habits to see real true change. I would meet with clients in my office three days a week to discuss how they were progressing on their weight loss plan. Yes, there was a sales component—we had numbers to hit—but I also knew I was helping people, and because of that belief, I was able to be successful in my position.

I remember Martha, who came in faithfully for every visit. She was probably 80 lbs. overweight and would lose 2 lbs. on Monday and gain 3lbs by Friday. She purchased everything we sold. She was a weight loss company's dream client. I think in her first year, she must have spent close to $10,000. When her first year was completed, it was required to meet with the client, and if they hadn't met their goal weight, to have them sign up for another year. I brought her into my office and took a seat alongside her.

"Martha, you know we all love you here, right? There's nothing more we want than to help you lose weight. I can't, in good conscience, ask you to pay thousands of dollars more when I believe you really need some professional help with this." I had printed a list of a few local overeaters anonymous group meetings. "Maybe try starting here."

Martha said. "I know I haven't lost weight, and I know it's expensive, but I love coming here. I feel so connected to everyone, and it's a place I feel safe where you won't judge me."

"Martha, you are welcome to come see us. However, everything you said is exactly what you would get going to these meetings. I will even go with you to your first meeting if you would like me to." *I would have been fired if the corporate office knew I was having this conversation, but I didn't care.* "Martha, You are a 60-year-old woman who goes to work Monday-Friday, goes home, and takes care of your disabled husband. You work hard for that money, and I think you're just lonely. We need to get you with a group of women who will support you, not enable you, and that's what it's going to be if we keep going. I can't do that because I care. Does that make sense?"

"Yes. Can I still stop in and see you once in a while, maybe on a Saturday?"

"Of course."

I went with Martha to her first meeting. I probably could have kept going for myself! It was a great place where people could share their stories. Everyone was extremely welcoming, and she liked hearing others relatable struggles with food. Martha stopped in once a month for the next six months. We always loved seeing her. She would bring us healthy recipes and gifts she made. Martha made a few new friends and began walking three times a week. She lost 10lbs. She was happy, and that made me happy.

CHAPTER 5: Opportunity Knocks

2005 I found a job online. It was listed as a Consultant position in Tampa, Florida. Base plus commission with a six-figure opportunity. Is this for real? Plastic Surgery, Fitness, Beauty, Weight loss experience a plus. Hmm, I want to make six figures. Maybe I'll apply for the heck of it. I landed an interview immediately and was scheduled to drive to Tampa for the interview. At the time, I was living in northern Florida and figured it would take me three hours. That morning, I got up, and it was torrential rain. If you happen to live in Florida or have experienced this rainfall, you know it's scary, like pull over to the side of the road because you can't see in front of you scary! I had to travel I-4, which is the most dangerous interstate in the country. Here's how the conversation went.

Me: I'm not going.

My now husband Mike: You need to go.

Me: I'm not—it's raining so hard.

Mike: Michelle, you will be fine. You have a great opportunity. Get in the car and go.

I called my parents and spoke with my father, who is also a coach.

Dad: Get in the car.

Me: I'm scared.

Dad: Of course, you are, now go.

Me: I can't.

Dad: You can, you will be fine.

My mom in the background: Honey, God's watching over you. I'll say a prayer.

Me: Fine. I'm going.

My interview lasted all of 30 minutes. I remember a beautiful, short-haired blond woman looking down at my resume. Not that it was crazy impressive. I had worked for an insurance company, a software company, and a weight loss company. I did include on my resume that I was a collegiate athlete. I always think that lets people know you have winning traits. At least it does for me. When I look at a resume, that's a reason to call. Teamwork, drive, work ethic, determination, the list goes on. The interview ended with the woman telling me I had the IT factor. "Well, thank you."

I didn't know exactly what she meant, but I was pretty confident she liked me. I made it out to the parking lot, and my phone rang.

"I'm offering you the job; it starts in two weeks. We will send all the information to your email and get your tickets to fly to Michigan. Are you in?"

"Oh, wow...um... Yes, I'm in."

* * *

It didn't take long to pack up, a few weeks later I've moved to Tampa, Florida, to start my new career as a Plastic Surgery Physician's Consultant. My first day on the job; I'm wearing my black, fitted dress I bought on sale at JC Penney and a pair of black heels which I must say we're quite cute. *I wish I still had those.* I've always been thankful I knew how to walk in heels properly. Being an athlete my entire life, I always cringe when I see the girl who's never quite comfortable. She has that awkward and clunky walk like she needs to get out of her heels and back into her tennis shoes (or called sneakers depending on where you live in the united states). I had it down, and with my fresh box of hair color and my new outfit, I was ready to schedule procedures.

My education on plastic surgery consisted of a weeklong training that covered the names of the procedures we offered and a brief explanation of how each procedure was performed. Each day after training, I went back to my hotel room (shout out to Drury Hotels, which was my home away from home for many years. No shout out from me on the powdered eggs—those are nasty). I studied—a lot. I was told I would have to present in front of the founder, Dr. David Kent. I hadn't spent time with a doctor apart from being sick. I didn't know any doctors personally, and figured I had to really pay attention, prove myself and stand out on everything I learned.

People say I'm the most competitive person they know. Yes, I do like to win, and I'm competitive with myself. It's an internal drive I've always had and want to do my best. I don't always succeed, but I always try. On the last day of training, I walked to the door, peeked my head in and slowly took a seat at one of the two maroon colored leather chairs in front of his desk. My palms were sweaty, and I was thinking, good thing I didn't write the answers on my palms or I definitely would have sweated them right off! Dr. Kent looked directly at me and asked me if I had studied. I responded quickly with "All night." I sat in front of him as he fired off questions. My voice was shaking, but I got through it and answered all the questions correct. I remember him smiling and saying, "Wow, you're going to be great, Michelle."

Those words of affirmation expanded my confidence, and I relied on him for many years to provide those same words to the hundreds of other consultants that worked for us. I was ready to meet with patients and had my consultation down. On my first day in the office, I scheduled seven new patients. By the end of my first week, Dr. Kent was calling the office to find out more about me.

What is a Lifestyle Lift?

If only I had a nickel for every time I was asked this question! Lifestyle Lift was a national facial cosmetic surgery practice. It wasn't a trademarked procedure—there's no such thing. Lifestyle Lift was a trademarked brand and offered facial rejuvenation procedures under local anesthesia.

If you took the time to go online to research, you would have found all kinds of different answers. Isn't that typical of the world we live in though? We are a country that's divided right down the middle in our beliefs, so why would it be any different no matter what the topic? Movies, restaurants, religion, politics, and yes-even plastic surgery, everyone has an opinion and you can argue both sides on any and all of it.

Your belief system is one of the strongest forces that affect the decisions you make. We accumulate our beliefs through what we hear, what we see, what we read, and essentially any external influence. The psychology behind why we make decisions and how we form our opinions is so fascinating to me, but let's stay focused on this topic. There's a well known in the industry website that provides a platform for consumers to ask questions to plastic surgeons, read reviews, etc.

"**RealSelf** is a resource for people considering cosmetic treatments and providers seeking to connect with them. We help millions of people find the right treatment and provider for them."[2] Online it states they are considered the Yelp of plastic surgery. If you keep googling, you then can find negative comments about them. The company was founded and initially self-funded in 2006 by a former male executive with a background in

---

[2] https://www.realself.com/plastic-surgery

technology. In 2018 the company received 40 million in funding.

The website brings millions of viewers each day from people both inside and outside the industry. They offer information free to consumers as well as medical professionals however you can upgrade to a paid membership. Medical professionals can buy the membership and buy advertising based on certain criteria. Now I don't work there, I don't even know anyone that works there. I'm sure they are all nice people. From what I can see it looks like they are doing some good things. What I would also say is that when someone invests 40 million dollars and scales a business, they are relying heavily on expected profits.

I make a point to mention that because I think people get too stuck on what they believe, again, what they see, what they hear, what they read. The question comes back to and what I get asked regularly; how does anyone know what to believe? What I know is that every day we are bombarded with information on the television, radio, magazines and Internet.

Anybody can build a website and put information up. You have to do your research from many sources when it comes to plastic surgery. There are pros and cons to everything. I'm sure RealSelf can be a good resource, and so is taking additional steps to cover all your bases.

Interestingly, when you google Lifestyle Lift, RealSelf pulls up first.

According to RealSelf, Lifestyle Lift was *a* term for a variety of facial-rejuvenation procedures offered at a cosmetic surgery chain *of the* same name. Founded in 2001 by ear, nose, and throat physician Dr. David Kent, the *Lifestyle Lift* Company promised quick, low-cost mini facelifts *and* other procedures, *with local anesthesia* and short recovery times. The information online goes on to say, the business operated in ways that raised many red flags. Here are a few:

- It offered physicians who weren't board-certified plastic surgeons the opportunity to perform plastic surgery.

- Doctors could be contractors and not full-time, accredited employees.
- Because the procedures were performed under local anesthesia, Lifestyle Lift practices weren't required to have a true surgical setup. They also weren't affiliated with any hospitals.
- Patients were offered deals if they confirmed their surgery dates within a few days of their consultations.
- Advertisements showed before and after photos with excellent results, but RealSelf member reviews and photos showed such issues as permanent disfigurement, scarring, pain, and unsatisfactory results.

Lifestyle Lift reflected a 70% worth it rating on this site. Back to the pros and cons, Lifestyle lift marketed to and provided cosmetic surgery options to the everyday person. The company brought a never-before-seen level of competition to the private practice physician, which led to a lot of bad blood and enemies. But just because they inserted some competition into the cosmetic surgery field didn't make them bad. There are plenty of great private practice surgeons I wouldn't send my enemy too. The best thing you can do for yourself, whether wanting a Lifestyle Lift type procedure or any surgical procedure, is to do all your research. Feel free to Internet search, (because unless you live off the grid in which case you're not reading this book about plastic surgery, you're going to start searching anyway), but please talk to the doctor directly—talk to real patients. Talk to a coach.

If you are having a cosmetic procedure, either major or minor, it's important to point out there are risks and the possibility of something going wrong. You have to be ready both physically and mentally. You make the choice, no one else. I mention it because no matter how great a surgeon, complications can occur, and you as the patient have to own that risk. You will hear me say throughout the book, "Know Before You Go!"

Some important questions to Ask:

1. How many of these types of procedures have you performed?
2. How many years have you been performing this type of procedure?
3. Do you specialize in any particular type of procedure or work primarily on certain areas of the body?
4. Am I a good candidate for this type of procedure?
5. What are your board certifications?
6. Is the procedure performed under local or general anesthesia, and why?
7. Is there any risk of complications from this procedure, and if so, what are they?
8. Do you have hospital privleges?
9. Can I see before and after photos?
10. Can you provide me with a patient I can speak directly to?

CHAPTER 6: My Oprah A-ha Moment

I was a few weeks into the job when Doris walked into my consultation room. Doris was a 67-year-old, petite woman with just above her shoulder's brown hair. She was wearing a blue cardigan set and khakis straight off the rack at Ann Taylor. She was warm and friendly, yet I immediately observed she was uncertain if she had made the right decision to come in.

"Hi, Doris, my name is Michelle. I'm your physician's consultant. It's so nice to meet you, thank you for coming in to see us today."

Since I was dealing with a much older population, I always incorporated addressing my age at the beginning of my consultations. I knew it was what most of the women, if not all, were thinking. I would be, so why not address it right from the start? I never wanted a patient to feel uncomfortable or think I was less than understanding because I was many years younger. I put it right out there and explained we are all on the same aging path just at different times.

Doris began sharing with me that after 45 years of marriage; her husband left her for a young woman. He cleared out the bank accounts, emptied his custom mahogany closets, leaving her a note on the kitchen counter. As you can imagine, Doris was devastated and left with a new world she didn't know.

Doris had been a stay at home mom her entire life. She had gone to college, yet married young and had her children. Her husband worked a good job, and they decided early on she would stay home to raise the boys. She raised her two sons, who, after college, moved to the west coast, and she didn't see them often. Doris said she had spent the previous six months trying to deal with the devastation that happened to her and it was time to do something for herself and make some life changes.

I thanked Doris for sharing her story and explained our procedures and doctors. Doris spent some time looking in the mirror, discussing her areas of concern, and then how we would be able to help her. We discussed risks, recovery, pricing, and selected her dates for pre-op to meet the doctor and procedure date. When we went to sign the paperwork, Doris seemed to hesitate.

"Do you have a question, Doris?"

"I don't know."

"What's going on?"

Doris paused, "I don't know... it's really a lot of money to spend. I don't know if I should do this. Maybe I'm crazy. I'm 67-years-old, I don't know if it's worth it."

I paused a minute and looked Doris right in the eyes.

"Doris, I'm going to say this to you because you've shared your personal story with me, so I hope you don't think this is too forward, however, I have to say it. You don't know if the procedure is worth it, or you don't know if you're worth it?"

Doris looked right back at me without blinking and said, "Let's do it."

Several months went by, and I had moved on to a new role within the organization. I had stopped into the Tampa office and was given a letter addressed to me. Doris had written me. As I started reading, I had to take a seat. Doris' words had brought me to tears. She stated she had gone through so much sadness over the last year, and she felt alone. She said it was such a big leap of faith, and since having the procedure; her entire life had turned around. Doris got her first job ever as a receptionist in a real estate office. She met a nice man online that had lost his spouse a few years back. She wrote beautifully about her new life and felt beautiful, alive and 20 years younger. She enclosed a picture of herself, and I immediately recognized she had updated her hair color and style and was wearing makeup. At the end of the letter, Doris wrote exactly this, and I remember it verbatim because it has always stayed with me:

"Words can never express my gratitude for pushing me outside my comfort zone. You took the time to hear my story and encouraged me to go for it. Thank you, Michelle, I am forever grateful."

At that very moment, I realized the real influence I had on being a part of changing someone's life. It wasn't about the number of procedures I scheduled—it was the ability to connect with someone in a way that can motivate and inspire them to do something better. It was the moment there was a shift in me from understanding; I'm not a salesperson. I'm a coach... I had the ability to do great things with my skills.

I don't know where Doris is—hopefully enjoying a mojito on a warm beach somewhere. I do know I've shared her story with hundreds of consultants because I believe it to be a powerful one, and it's what keeps my love affair ongoing with this industry.

CHAPTER 7: Adult Education

In 2012, I worked for a company that provided full-body plastic surgery. We had multiple locations and some incredibly, experienced plastic surgeons who had seen it all. During my time, if I wasn't working with a consultant or patient, you could find me in the Exam or Operating Room.

The patient and I both signed informed consent, and I was in full scrubs in case anyone was concerned with why I would be in the room. Patients' family members always ask if they can watch. However, there are strict HIPAA regulations, so the answer is no.

I observed hundreds of doctor consultations and surgeries too, hanging on every word, eyes wide open. I would see women coming in who had breast implants that had ruptured, college girls wanting their noses fixed, men looking for calf implants—you name it, we saw it. You can't get this experience in a textbook. No way. This was medical education at its finest, and I loved every minute of it.

My client, Lilah, never knew what it felt like to really like her body. She told me she had a hard time looking back at photos of herself. Lilah lost her mother at the age of five and was raised by her brothers and father, who loved her very much but didn't know too much about what a girl needed.

Lilah had friends and learned from them most of what she said she needed to know, and thankfully, a grandma who could give her some advice from time to time. Still, Lilah said she had a weight problem from a very young age, and it continued to escalate as a grown woman. Lilah said she threw herself into her schoolwork and went on to become an educator in the public schools. This is where she met her husband John, who too struggled with his weight but not to the degree Lilah had. Lilah said she never had a problem with dating, although looking back, she said it was likely because she was somewhat as she stated, "promiscuous." She was also fortunate to not go through too much bullying in school. Her older brothers were very popular, and being from a small town, nobody wanted to mess with her.

Lilah said her weight gain was slow and steady until she became pregnant with her daughter. She packed on another 70lbs quickly, and after the baby, she couldn't take the weight off. Lilah and John tried to have more children, but she couldn't get pregnant. She knew it was because of the extra weight she was carrying, and so after many failed diet attempts, she decided to have bariatric surgery.

Over the next five years, Lilah shed all the baby weight and another 80 lbs. and she had maintained that weight loss for several years. This was when I met Lilah. A woman, who to look at, dressed seemed to anyone from the outside what you would call normal weight range. It was when Lilah got undressed that her story unfolded.

Lilah was carrying around extra skin on all areas of her body. A lot of it.

"I look in the mirror, and I'm not any happier than I was fat."

"First of all, Lilah, look at the accomplishment of your weight loss! Second, you are only halfway through your journey. You're here because you know that it's time to complete your transformation, right? This isn't a race, what's most important to you?"

"My stomach and back, then my arms."

"OK, let's start there."

We talked about the surgeries in great length, as each one was a major operation. Lilah was in good health, thankfully, so we were confident together the doctor would clear her. Lilah met with the doctor, and they discussed her first surgery would consist of a circumferential incision (around her body) to remove the belt of excess skin and fat. This is known as a lower body lift. Also, the doctor would be completing a traditional brachioplasty (arm lift). He talked about potentially doing a breast lift as well.

Lilah stated that wasn't an area that bothered her, and, in her words, "I think my boobs held up pretty well."

After the visit with the surgeon and nurse to cover all other pertinent information, we had a conversation about what to expect both physically and emotionally. As a Coach, I knew that Lilah was going to need a lot of support, as this was a much longer recovery process than other procedures. We discussed having her procedure over her summer break. Since John worked in the school system as well, he would be able to take care of her and her daughter.

Lilah started with a full-body lift. Money wasn't an issue as she had inherited money when she turned 18. She said it had to do with the death of her mother, but I didn't press it as I could see her eyes well up with the mention of her mom's name. I asked Lilah if she shared with her family outside of John that she would be having surgery, and she said yes, they would all be there at the hospital. Well, that's awesome.

Both her brothers were married with big families. She said she felt so blessed to have the support of her family. I was honored to be a part of her journey. I called Lilah the night before, as I did with almost all the patients I coach. She said she was nervous, excited, and anxious. I told her those were all normal emotions, and we said a prayer together on the phone. This would likely be against most corporate rules, but since we were writing the rules, I didn't care. Quite frankly, even if I weren't writing the rules, I would have broken it for prayer.

The next day, Lilah had her procedure followed by her second procedure the following month. It wasn't an easy recovery. Lilah said it was a lot more painful than expected, but now years later, she would tell you it reminded her of having a baby. The pain you go through was awful, but now she can't remember anything other than in her words, "That nasty flabby skin is gone and I look good."

Lilah and I stayed in touch for about a year after her procedures. She looked amazing, and she felt amazing! She was happy, and you could tell. The journey started in a place of sadness and is now in a place of happiness. While the journey is always ongoing as self-improvement is, she feels good, and that is beautiful.

According to the American Society of Plastic Surgery:

A **body lift** improves the shape and tone of the underlying tissue that supports skin and fat. Excess sagging skin and fat are removed, and the procedure(s) can improve a dimpled, irregular skin surface.[3]

Wikipedia's definition of a **Brachioplasty**, commonly called an arm lift, is a surgical procedure to reshape and provide improved contour to the upper arms and connecting area of the chest wall. While "brachioplasty" is commonly used to describe a specific procedure for the upper arms, the term can also be used to describe any surgical arm contouring. Brachioplasty is often used to address

---

[3]https://www.plasticsurgery.org/cosmetic-procedures/arm-lift

issues such as excessive loose skin or excessive fat in the arms when it does not respond well to diet and exercise.[4]

If you are someone who has experienced dramatic weight loss, you may want to undergo body lift surgery. It is a very complex procedure, so you need to meet certain criteria to be eligible. Here are a few things that may consider you a good candidate for body lift surgery:

- Lost a significant amount of weight
- Have droopy skin, tissue, and fat around your abdomen
- Weight has been stable for a few years. Most plastic surgeons recommend waiting approximately two years to avoid fluctuation and avoid regaining weight loss
- Good health
- Do not plan on becoming pregnant after surgery
- Have realistic expectations

[4] https://en.wikipedia.org/wiki/Brachioplasty

CHAPTER 8: Winners Win

I was training all Patient Consultants at Lifestyle Lift in 2006. I think we had 10 or 11 locations then. I would fly in to work one on one with a consultant and observe their consultation to help them improve. We didn't have a strong formal training process, so I created one. Years later, I did receive my training certification. However, when we developed the curriculum, it was a combination of what they had been teaching and everything I had learned from my years in weight loss. I didn't see much difference between the two in terms of consultation. I understood the risks were higher, but the emotion behind it was all the same.

I was one on one, getting to talk intimately with someone about an aesthetic they wanted to change. We could help them and so let's help them. What's so hard about that? Why, if someone came to us for help, and we could help them, would we let them walk out? I trained this way and promoted that message to everyone because I believed wholeheartedly in it. I've spent the majority of my life in a leadership role. My California business partner says I can't help it because I'm a Leo and a double fire sign. Whatever that means!

It's not always easy being the boss. You can't always expect everyone to like you, but I always make sure to be true to what I believe is the right thing. My dad always says integrity is doing the right thing when no one is watching. I can hear his words to me from coaching me growing up that still rings true in business, "Keep your head in the game, Michelle. Hustle. Don't take your eye off the ball—stay in it."

I've never understood how someone moves up the ladder, or as the business world calls it, sits up in their ivory tower, why they would want to become disconnected to the business. I have found from my experience many corporate people spend all their time looking at spreadsheets and have no idea what's going on inside the business. Why do you think television shows like *Undercover Boss* become popular? It's because there's a story behind every employee and a different perspective of the business that you will never see from the tower. My advice to any business leaders who may be reading my book, get on the field, and play in the game. You'll have a much better chance of winning.

I remember Dr. Kent asking me to lunch in 2007 to discuss more responsibility. I had covered the sales team regionally, and he wanted to know how I could handle running the offices nationally. He asked me how I would build a national team.

"Having played sports my whole life and the fact that we're having lunch at a lovely sports bar establishment, I would say this. Just like any great coach, if I am building a team, and I think of it like I'm going to the World Series, whom would I want out on the field? I want all-stars. I want great attitudes and people with skills, who play with heart and soul. I want people who can win. You can't win championships unless you have a strong team, and that's what I'm always working to build. If there's a player on the field who is struggling, we either coach them up or out. It's how I lead.

He said, "I love it. I know you can handle it."

I've seen quite a few all-stars in my career, all of which have gone on to do great things. It's amazing when you see talent. As a coach, you feel a sense of pride one, getting to coach them, and two, being part of their journey. Yes, it's business, but it's all the same.

I remember hiring this dynamic individual. It was the first time I truly understood the "IT" factor. She exuded energy like it was coming from her pores. Wow, who wouldn't want to be around this person? Her light shined bright, and she wasn't dulling it for anyone. I mentioned earlier, or somewhere in this book, about having to be resilient. We hear the word 'NO' a lot. We also spend a lot of time with inconsistent people, procrastinators, or sometimes in an unhappy place in their life. This young woman was never pacified. She uplifted, never wavered, and it was contagious. She was a winner, and I was honored to work with her.

I can't write a book without mentioning another all-star. She ran circles around the rest. She was the captain of the team without the title. I didn't have to ask; I could tell within five minutes of meeting her. She was up against challenges, and she worked through them. She praised her team members when they did well. She showed up and played even harder under the spotlight. I nicknamed her my Derek Jeter (in case you live in a cave, Derek Jeter played shortstop for the Yankees and is ranked as one of the great players of all time). We both moved on from our positions, worked for a short while at another company, and, hopefully, will work together again. She's moved on in different leadership positions and will continue to find professional success. Again, another winner.

You have winners, and you have learners. And with people comes drama. I always tried to shield the team from the behind the scenes problems just like parents fighting behind closed doors. My job was to keep people motivated and in a focused, positive state. I'm a coach. I'm in a meeting, and someone's talking about how someone should be fired.

"She's terrible." What? I can fix this. Let me work with her. Let me get this woman 20 years older than me to listen to what I have to say, to get her back on track."

I fly into her city, and she knows I'm coming. I never did surprise visits—it wasn't my management style. I approach my coaching the same way I meet with patients. Let's get real. Talk to me. I sit down in the worn white pleather chair. She sits across from me and puts her head down. She sees the report, and she knows what this conversation looks like, at least what she's expecting. I say her name. We lock eyes.

"Brenda, what I want to do today is find out what you believe is working well and what areas you see that we can improve on. I'm going to observe two consultations then we will come back into this room and review together. My job is to support you and provide you the tools to be a great patient consultant. I know you bring years of professional experience, so I am confident this will be an easy adjustment. You have to trust I'm going to do what I can, and I need the same from you. Does that work? Great! Tomorrow I will have you observe me, and we can take turns meeting with patients. We can ask the patients about their experience as well."

We start with her beliefs.

"What do you think of the role of a Patient Coordinator? What do you believe about the doctors? What about the patients?"

Ding! Ding! Ding! And there it is!

"These patients have no money. Why would I run credit when they probably don't have credit? The last patient I met with works at the mall food court, she can't afford plastic surgery. These are not the people that I expected would be coming in for plastic surgery. They can't afford it."

I'm thinking, 'wow, that's so rude, but I know she's just frustrated.'

You have to understand in a sales job you hear the word *No* more often than you hear yes. You have people come to meet with you just for something to do. If you're not centered and resilient and optimistic, you won't make it in any sales job.

"Thank you for sharing your beliefs, Brenda. Now we know what we have to work through. Do you believe these patients want to look and feel better about themselves?"

"Yes."

"Ok, they deserve to have something done for themselves?"

"Yes."

"Do you believe if a patient meets with you and presents something about themselves they don't like or want to change, that your job is to help them get to a place of confidence?"

"Yes."

"Ok, now let me ask you this, Brenda. Are you turning over every stone and providing these patients with every possible solution that could help them reach their goals?"

Brenda's head dropped, "No, Probably not. But they don't have money."

"They don't have *EASY* money. They don't have good credit or a credit card, but don't sell anyone short, Brenda. You can't do that. I don't want you to feel bad. I know you are a caring person and took this position because you want to help people and make a difference, right?"

"Yes."

"Ok, then let's go through every way possible—what questions to ask, what solutions we can extend these patients. Here's the difference between us and maybe a private practice. When a potential patient sets an appointment at a plastic surgeon's office, they likely have the affordable means to move forward.

In fact, many surgeons charge a fee for a consultation, which includes meeting the doctor. Our potential patients received a free consultation and meet with you, and most often not the doctor unless he's out of surgery or between patient visits, right? If we saw the typical plastic surgery patients, they wouldn't necessarily be coming in to meet with us.

A large demographic of cosmetic patients, which is typically our demographic, are middle to even lower income. They want to look good too and want a procedure that's affordable. They may have the funds or may not know how to come up with the money, but trust me when I say, they will. Some people take out loans, save up, borrow, dip into retirement funds, and 401K. You name it, they will find it. Women are the most resourceful. We find ways to make things happen. It's in our genes.

Now, some of the people you meet with may need ideas, and that's where you step in. Let's write down all the ways someone could come up with additional funds. We have to help the people coming to see us, and we also can't prejudge. You never know someone's financial situation. I know plenty of people who live in a mansion with no furniture and other people who live in a trailer and stash thousands under their mattress. Don't fall into the trap of thinking you know, or putting your feelings and beliefs on that person sitting in front of you. Give them every opportunity. Can you commit to doing that?"

"Yes."

Brenda worked for the company for four years. She was promoted twice.

CHAPTER 9: Discovery

I've always been curious. How can others not fascinate you? We are all so different and have unique stories. I've spent years observing and coaching both women and men. Men's decision-making style, from my experience, is simple, quick, and easy.

"I got these love handles here..." lifting his shirt, "I can't get rid of. I work out 5-6 days a week. Can you get rid of them?"

I laugh out loud. "I believe we can help you.

There you have it. Problem-Solution. For women, it's all about the journey, for men—they are on a mission. I did a study years ago—not a scientific study, but a 3-ring notebook with some chicken scratch notes. I followed consultation times of 75 women and 25 men. The average consultation time of an initial plastic surgery consultation (just with me) took a little under an hour. Men 23 minutes. No need for an entire book on it, short and sweet.

They say men buy and women shop. Lord knows we think differently, and we certainly buy differently. Women want to be taken on the journey. When I train and coach consultants, I always talk about not rushing the consultation. Take them out for dinner and drinks first, a little wine and dine—a little romance. With men, maybe not skip the drinks but all the rest of it, most of the time, they could skip it all.

It's right-brain, left-brain, emotion vs. logic, and with an industry that's predominately women; it's exactly why women professionals should be heavily represented in the aesthetic market. Not just as mid-level employees, but as executives—the decision-makers running the show. When it comes to all the ladies....all the single ladies, all the single ladies... who doesn't love a Beyoncé song? Sorry, quick break out in song distraction... not just single ladies, all ladies, we see a much more emotional and vulnerable side. It doesn't always start that way, but it gets there.

Because I'm not interested in surface conversation, let's get down to the truth. The real you—not the 'you' in social circles. I want to talk to you. I want to talk to the girl who was teased in middle school for her big nose. And the woman who skips the pool with her kids because she's embarrassed to be seen in a bathing suit. The secret she's been hiding and covering up. Take the mask off in this room, please; because that's the only way I can help you. I know it's not easy to trust someone you just met, but in this room, there's no judgment, no bias. For all you moms of little girls, out-sing with me a frozen favorite... LET it GO! I promise to listen and feel it right there with you.

A psychologist would call me an empath, a person who feels the happiness and sadness of others. I call it my superpower and God-given talent. As a plastic surgery coach, I dig in. I love asking questions because people are fascinating, and questions lead to the real. One of my favorite questions to ask in a consultation is, "What do you want for yourself?"

Working with women and hearing so many stories, there's a common theme. People care way too much about what other people want and what other people think. We live in a superficial world full of judgment—a world of filters and staged photos. Look at my Facebook profile. In my perfectly angled, after ten takes later, photo. It's ok but come on ladies. Is this a secret to anyone? Pull every phone over the age of 16, and you will most likely find some type of face/body altering app. If it's not an app, it's a filter.

My bathroom lights are so bright I scare myself in the morning. Woah, I look rough! Where did those bags under my eyes come from? I need a trip to Home Depot® to get some better lighting in here, but for now, let me turn some off. Yes, that's right. I get ready with mood lighting. Not too dark, not too bright lighting; it's my filter! Yes, it's awful. As a mom, I don't want my daughter to feel like she has to alter herself. The only way we can work through this is to talk about it because getting older and seeing changes isn't always easy.

I have met with thousands of women over 50 that make the same statement, verbatim. "I look in the mirror, and I don't recognize myself anymore." They tell me that they still feel like that young girl inside, but the outside no longer matches the inside. Only now, as I get closer to approaching 50, do I fully understand that feeling.

This story is always funny to me. When I started at Lifestyle Lift, I was 29-years-old. We only offered facial rejuvenation, so the women I consulted with were much older. They would look at me and say, "Oh honey, what do you know? Look how young you are." Now fast forward the clock. Now I get asked all the time when I do a facial rejuvenation consultation, "Have you had it done?" And there you have it. No love for father time when it comes to wrinkles and frown lines!

So, let's get real, Dr. Phil real. Not the surface, but the real-real. Plastic Surgery can be awesome and life changing. I could go on about all of the life changing experiences I've been a part of, but there is a 'but,' and I don't mean a tiny waist with a disproportionate kind of butt. I'm trying to say that if there is something about you that you deeply believe, think, and feel would present a better you, a more confident you, and you've weighed the risk/reward, than YOU, my friend, go for it. Not for him, not for them, or anybody but you! Who cares what people think? Be real, be you, and own it.

Everyone has an opinion—people judge, and just like I tell my daughter, the best thing you can do is worry about yourself because, trust me, those people judging and giving their opinions are dealing with their own set of internal issues. Look at the Kardashian's, these are beautiful women who have been placed under the highest level of scrutiny. They have been judged more than any other women, probably in the world. I don't walk in their Jimmy Choo™ stilettos or Yeezy™ sneakers, but I'm certain that they have deep-rooted insecurities like everyone else.

These women have access to every possible procedure and service. They are real-life marketing dolls. I can't blame them for taking advantage of what's out there. Ask yourself if a plastic or cosmetic surgeon said they could help you get rid of cellulite; would you try it? A lot of what they've also had are non-surgical procedures and treatments, many of which they promote on the shows, which then provides those doctors "celebrity status."

So back to my point, enough with the surface, share your story and let me help educate you and uplift you. Get you to a place where you are feeling yourself, and if that means choosing to have cosmetic surgery, make sure it's what you want. My take away: Do You Boo!

CHAPTER 10: Patient Stories

Good to Grave

70-year-old Amelia said she was determined to look good until the Lord laid her to rest. Amelia didn't look her age. She spent years wearing sunscreen and large brim hats to protect her skin. I asked her to remove her neck scarf so I could take a look. She laughed.

"I live in a scarf!" Replied Amelia.

"It's 85 degrees outside. I hope we can get you out of these!"

Her skin had some laxity. She was a fairly thin woman, and these are her words, not mine! Amelia was on a fixed income. She lived in a small ranch style home that she had paid off years ago. She said she bought it in 1976 for $26,000. She'd been living on her retirement pension and social security. She said her son had used her to cosign a loan and had screwed up her credit a little. We ran it to see what we could get. She was approved for $2500. Amelia smiled immediately and said, “Great, I’ll do the rest on layaway.”

My experience with layaway was every summer from 1979-1983. My mom would take us to Hills Department Store to pick out clothes, and we would stop in each week to chip away at the balance. And that’s exactly what Amelia did. She faithfully sent us a check for $200 every month until her balance was paid off. The day she arrived for her pre-op visit with the doctor, we celebrated with a cake with her name on it. She was our first every plastic surgery layaway, and she doesn’t know it, but she paved the way for thousands more because people still do payment plans to this day.

Gucci Anyone?

If anyone has worked in south Florida, you know it can be different. Miami has the most plastic surgeons and procedures anywhere in the United States. The competition is fierce, and it’s probably the closest I got in my career to Let’s Make a Deal.

Some offices in Miami, it's all about the best price. And while there are great doctors, you can find some unqualified docs, and some ridiculously cheap surgeries too. If you research the number of deaths in plastic surgery, a Miami story will most likely pop up. At Lifestyle Lift, the South Florida office was like nowhere else. I met Marianna on a Thursday. She was a beautiful Hispanic woman with long black hair and big brown eyes. She told me right away she had gone to four different consultations and would make her decision based on what we charged her, and if we could do her procedure by the end of the week. This wasn't uncommon, patients wanting a deal and procedure right away.

We had Marianna meet the doctor, and after her medical evaluation, it was determined we could get her on the schedule for Friday. We had been open in the new location for a few months and had struggled to get surgeries on the schedule. They flew me in to see what was going on. Marianna wanted to pay cash for the procedure and plunked down

$4,000. Based on the prices back then, she was a bit short. She went from arguing with me to practically crying because she wanted the procedure badly. She said she was getting remarried in a month, and her hot, Latin boyfriend was 20 years younger.

"Well, let's figure this out. We have to get you looking hot."

Through our conversation, Marianna shared with me she sold purses, and would just need to sell a few more to get the remaining money.

"What kind of purses?" I asked.

"Gucci and a few Louis Vuitton bags."

"Wait. What? You have them in your car?"

"Yes, in my trunk."

"Can you go get them; I may have some customers?"

Marianna went down to her trunk while I talked to the team.

"Ok, ladies, I don't know if they are real, or hot, or what, but the patient I'm with sells purses. She is getting them out of her trunk, and I'm buying one. Who's in?"

Marianna came back and proceeded to spread her bags throughout the lobby on chairs and coffee tables. Back then; it wasn't uncommon to have twenty people in the lobby. I told Mariana, "We don't normally do this, but today we're having a purse party." And so, for the next four hours, Marianna proceeded to sell twelve handbags, including three to the staff. She made money for her procedure and enough to add her upper eyes. I'm not sure that was the most ethical way to get a patient scheduled, but we had fun doing it. Marianna looked fabulous for her wedding, and we got an amazing deal on a designer handbag.

It's A Party

Standing room only. Every chair was filled, and you would have thought we were wearing roller skates. There was always a crazy buzz and momentum when we opened new locations. We went all out, making sure we created a Grand Opening, but this particular office was the craziest of them all. We hadn't anticipated such a crazy opening day. However, at the time, we were running national TV commercials and had locations in the same territory, so we couldn't have planned for the anticipation for our arrival.

My colleagues and I had flown out a week early to get the office properly set up and make sure all processes, procedures, and staff were in place. There was always a lot of attention around the launch of a new location. There were also a lot of expenses tied to the success of a new center, so we decided we would be all-hands-on-deck. I remember saying to our call center director, fill the schedule, we've got this!

We opened the doors at 9 am for the first consultation. By noon, we had seen twelve patients. By 3 pm, twenty-five, and by the end of the day, we finished with forty-seven new consultations and had scheduled forty-three of them. For anyone reading this who has done consultations, your eyebrow is raised, and mouth is dropped open. This wasn't an open house. These were scheduled appointments, one-on-ones.

They were coming in droves, and the day was a blur. I remember telling one of our team members to order food, cookies, drinks, and call cabs because we are keeping this party going (no such thing as Uber back then). When we finished that night, I remember my colleague and I slouching in our chairs, taking our heels off, and looking at each other like, "what just happened?" It was 10 pm on the East Coast. We called corporate to let them know their opening was a huge success. Now we had to do that again tomorrow.

The Laugh Factory

Quick true story. She walks in my office, tells her young daughter to have a seat, and quickly pulls down her yoga pants and thong.

"What can you do for me?"

I laughed out loud. "Well, this isn't usually how the consultation goes, but tell me, what's bothering you?"

I'm trying to ignore the fact that I know this person; she's a bit of a celebrity, and she's comfortable enough to flash me her privates. People never cease to surprise me.

"Ok, let's talk."

From Galas to Garage Sales

We pull up to the valet, and I notice it looks like a scene from a movie. I'm attending a cancer research gala this evening for my husband's job. We have a table with what you could say are high rollers. I say this because, during the gala, it comes time for the auction where bidding starts at $5k. The woman next to me leans over and tells me that last year, she and her husband won the African safari trip. I look over at him, and he's already three Dewar's and waters in. I don't think he cares what she bids on. I look over at Mike, "We are not bidding on that. I know it's for a good cause, but these people are competing—all for winning—let them go at it. I'm listening to these bids, and they are up to $100,000. I'm seeing paddles going up like nobody's business. Rich people don't play! Mike and I take a casual stroll over to the silent auction table and bid on the dinner for two at Morton's Steak House, and we laugh to each other.

"I love steak."

"Me too

The next morning, I had to be at work at 9 am. I didn't get home until midnight, and for me, that's hours past my bedtime. I dragged myself into work, unlike me, which is why I go to bed early. I'm tired, but it's game time. That's how I always approached my day doing consultations. Show up to play. Attitude in check, smile on my face, and ready to engage with people who need me. It may sound cheesy to some, but it's how I like to approach the job.

I always start the day looking in my car visor mirror, telling myself, "Today will be a great day." I laugh, close the mirror, flip it back up and get moving. The magic happens when the heels go on. My ladies know what I'm talking about. A lot of us go into work with flats but slip on the heels for some extra power. I freshen up in the mirror. I'm rockin' the leftover make-up from the gala. Every woman knows that a smoky eye looks better the next day.

My first consultation shows up. Shonda was a 30-year-old woman with a small frame. She has no idea how much this costs, but she saw the commercial and said she needed to get rid of her muffin top. We go through the full consultation, and she appears to be a good candidate. She tells me that she made some money from her big garage sale last weekend. I'm thinking to myself I really live in bizarro world. Can you imagine the women from last night's gala wearing Bergdorf Goodman's gowns and Christian Louboutins™, telling me they made money off a garage sale? She pulls a wad of money out of her bag and spreads it out on the coffee table.

"Wow, you are carrying all that around?"

She replies, "I want you to have it. If I keep it any longer, I will spend it on something else, and I really want this procedure. How much does that cover?"

How much did you make? Hmm, I really need to think about having a garage sale!”

“I sold everything. I moved out of the house, plus I had saved up some money, so there’s $3000 dollars there. Can you do it for that, it’s all I have?”

“Do you have money to live on?”

Not a lot, but I’ll be okay. My sister can help.”

I excuse myself and see if the doctor is free. He comes in and meets with Shonda. She is a good candidate and only needs one area of liposuction. She tells us she’s free anytime, and we look at the schedule to see if there’s an opening in a few days. No health issues, her sister can be her transportation and stay with her overnight. All the boxes are checked; let’s get her scheduled. I tell the doctor about her situation. We are in agreement; I go back and tell Shonda she doesn’t have to spend all her money, and she can pocket some. She stands up and hugs me.

“Thank you. I’m so excited!!”

“So are we, Shonda.”

I'd Do Anything

It's Monday morning, and I'm in the office. My Consultant partner is hungover from the night before and has no interest in seeing patients.

"Please, Michelle, I'm totally hungover. I went out with this guy last night..."

"Say no more. I want details later. I got ya, girl."

First up, Rayan. Rayan is a 29-year-old woman who tells me in the first two minutes of meeting that she wants to look like Beyoncé. I respond with, "Um, Don't we all?" I ask Rayan specific questions about her background and why she wants something now. She tells me her boyfriend is getting out of jail in two months, and she wants to be "lookin' good" when he sees her.

"OK!"

I ask Rayan about the areas she wants addressed, medical history, time off, budget with which she states she can pay all cash today.

"What do you do for work?"

"I'm a waitress at a club."

I'm certain Rayan is doing more than waiting tables, but it's none of my business other than the fact that I want to know more about her. I follow up with, "Which club do you work at?" Yep, that's a strip club right down the street.

"Do you dance as well?"

"Sometimes, I do. I do what I need too."

I respond with, "I'm not mad at ya. And so, we need to get you in and enough time to be healed and looking and feeling good. You have no medical issues, don't smoke, blood pressure is good, let's talk about weight."

"I smoke weed."

"OK, stop that for two weeks. Based on your height and weight, your Body Mass Index falls into the overweight category. Liposuction is not a weight loss procedure; however, it can help provide a nice contour. It's recommended patients are in the healthy BMI range, but that doesn't mean you can't still have the procedure and see a great result."

I get it, "I've tried to lose weight so many times. It's not happening, and I don't want to wait any longer."

I get Rayan set up with the doctor, and based on what we can get done, it would be in two procedures.

"One in two weeks if you stop the herb."

"I can."

"OK, good, the second procedure two weeks following. The total is $14,000."

"Dang, for real? OK, I'm $3K short. I can give you $11,000 right now and get the rest by Friday."

"Do you want to apply for financing?"

"I can't get credit, but I can get cash. I just need to turn a couple tricks."

I pause and ask myself if I should keep prying and ultimately decide not to touch that. Stone-faced, I respond with, "See you Friday afternoon then."

Rayan showed up Friday right before we closed, brought us the remaining balance, and had her procedures as scheduled. She looked great and sent us a picture of her in her tight hot pink spandex dress with her no longer incarcerated man by her side. Good Stuff.

Boobs Are Bad

Matt was 20-years-old. I couldn't help but notice his good looks when I walked over to introduce myself. He had big blue eyes and a beautiful smile. I walked alongside him down the hallway to the consultation room, making small talk to get a gauge on his personality. Matt walked with his head down, and when I asked him a question, he responded with, "Yes, ma'am..." Well, dang, I'm old. Anyway, Matt sat down, and I told him what we would be doing today. Our system gives us some data on potential patients, and I could see that Matt had made three previous appointments and never showed up. When I see this, I know there's a fear roadblock.

"I'm really glad you decided to come in today, Matt. My job is to help you. Everyone who walks through those doors has their own insecurities. I'm sure you were nervous coming in, and you're here, so congrats on taking that first step. I want you to know you can feel comfortable discussing your areas of concern. There's nothing weird or shameful, and there's no judgment. So, while I know it may feel uncomfortable being a young guy, it's ok; we have seen thousands of men your age. Would you mind sharing a bit of your story with me?"

Matt proceeded to tell me that he has been wearing a girdle under his shirts his entire life. He was ashamed of his body and did everything he could to hide his secret. He had avoided parties, swimming, and even being intimate with a girl. He said he managed to escape his teenage years of being bullied by avoiding a lot of interaction. He said he lived his life behind a computer. His younger sister convinced him to make an appointment with another plastic surgeon, but he never showed up for three different appointments he had made the last two years. My heart went out to him, and at the same time, I was jumping through the roof to think about how amazing he will look and feel.

"I can't imagine how difficult it's been for you. But here's the thing—you've spent your entire life focusing on this. Let's start focusing on the change. Deal? Now you made 3 appointments and never made it through the door. What made you say today's the day?"

"I met a girl online, and she wants to meet. I really like her."

"When are you meeting?"

"She will be home from college next month."

"Ok, then we need to schedule you right away. Our schedule is booked. However, I will find you a spot, I promise."

I immediately shared Matt's story with the doctor, and he agreed to fit him in. Matt had gynecomastia, which is excess fatty breast tissue; in layman's terms, he had man boobs. They were quite pronounced, and I could understand why he stayed covered up. Kids can be mean and hurtful, but all those years living like that—seriously heartbreaking.

We got Matt squared away, and I came in early the day of his procedure to be there.

I'm so excited I can't stand it! Matt smiled. "Seriously, I'm afraid for you." He looked at me. "You are ridiculously good-looking, smart, nice, and you are about to get rid of this shield that's been covering you for so long. Are you ready for this?"

"I am."

Matt's mom had been parking the car and made her way in. She gave Matt a hug, and the nurse took him back.

"Hi, you must be Matt's mother."

"Yes, I am."

"My name's Michelle. I met with Matt when he came in for his consultation. What a great son you've raised."

Matt's mom grabbed me and hugged me. "Would you like to sit and chat for a minute?"

"That would be great."

For the next hour, Matt's mom broke down that she didn't know how bad it was. She knew he was a bit of a loner but thought that was just who he was. She said she blamed herself, and she would have helped him earlier.

"You didn't know, and you can't blame yourself."

As a parent, I get it—nobody wants to see his or her child in pain.

"Here's the thing, it's done. Ok? He is in great hands, and he is removing this burden, so be proud that he's doing something about it. The worst thing you can do is sit and dwell. He doesn't blame you. He was great at hiding it, and plus what young boy wants to talk to his mom about boobs?"

She laughed. I called Matt after his procedure and was waiting for him at his 30-day pre-op. I think I was strangely more excited than he was. I hadn't met this kid before his consult, but I connected with him and his personal story. I wanted to coach him. Let me put this out there... he walked in with a fitted shirt on.

"What? Stop it!" I fell to the ground. He laughed. "No, you do not look this good! Tell me everything.

"Well, I met that girl online... an... and I met two others."

"Oh Lord! We've created a monster!"

Matt looked incredible, and better yet, he felt incredible. The doctor had changed his life, and the fact that I got to be a part of this awesome transformation, I'll never forget it.

What is Gynecomastia?

Gynecomastia is a condition of overdeveloped or enlarged breasts in men that can occur at any age. The condition can be the result of hormonal changes, heredity, obesity, or the use of certain drugs.

Gynecomastia can cause emotional discomfort and impair your self-confidence. Some men may even avoid certain physical activities and intimacy simply to hide their condition.

Gynecomastia is characterized by:

- Excess localized fat
- Excess glandular tissue development

- Sometimes excess breast skin
- Presence unilaterally (one breast) or bilaterally (both breasts)[5]

---

[5]https://www.plasticsurgery.org/cosmetic-procedures/gynecomastia-surgery

Chapter 11: You're So Vain

It's shallow, it's dangerous, it's lying, cheating... They must be insecure, shallow, narcissistic, selfish. "Did I miss anything?"

The term plastic surgery comes from the Greek work *plastikos*, which is to shape or mold. For the record Plastic Surgery can be divided into two categories; Reconstructive, which is performed to restore the form and function of a defect on the body.

Most people are familiar with breast reconstruction after a mastectomy or a child born with a cleft palate. These are considered to many acceptable forms of Plastic Surgery.

The second category is what we know to be called cosmetic surgery. Cosmetic Surgery is performed to augment otherwise healthy tissues to improve the appearance. For example, a tummy tuck or facelift. There are procedures that may fall somewhere in the middle however these are the two categories that essentially are done to make someone look more aesthetically pleasing. The question becomes is one good and the other bad?

My personal argument to the naysayers is this; if morality is up for discussion and someone considers it immoral, then the same would hold true for anything used to alter one's appearance, right? Piercing your ears, getting a tattoo, coloring your hair, or wearing make-up. I personally believe a lot has to do with our own personal motivations for pursuing a cosmetic procedure that has an impact on the ethics of the act itself. People do all kinds of things to make themselves look more attractive.

Do you want to have a conversation on morality with a 22-year-old girl sitting in front of you that tells you she has been picked on since the second grade about her big nose? Who spent most of her teen years crying because she hated looking in the mirror? Whose parents told her she needed to just deal with it, accept her looks and who sent her to a therapist when she turned fifteen. Who tells you she's always dated "down" because she felt safer and more secure with someone that she knew wasn't whom she truly wanted to be with? Who tells you she feels confident in everything else in her life but wants to make this one change because she believes for her, it is the right thing to do, is that immoral?

Self-love comes in different forms; so, for all you nose snubbers and people sitting on your high horse of morality, I say, get a life. Debate it all you like, I believe that helping a person participate in society in a much happier place is moral, ethical and beautiful. So there.

CHAPTER 12: Fake News

It's 2009; Lifestyle Lift is getting blasted with negative reviews. How is that possible? I'm traveling from city to city, and we have so many happy patients. Let's be clear—not everyone had the 5-star experience. However, our team was always, and I mean, always working toward delivering one. We were completely dedicated to how we could make things better and improve the patient experience. And then, one day, a colossal mistake.

A colleague, who I know to be a good guy, made a bad judgment call. I don't believe he was the sole driver, but he took the fall, and we all took a tumble. I'm not making excuses for him, but that was over ten years ago, and the Internet is a lot different now than it was then. Nobody really knew how to control what was put out there. Still, it was wrong, and the company paid the price—a lot more than a monetary fine.

It was like the words he spoke were said at a very slow warped speed. It was noon on Wednesday. We were conducting our usual national sales call where we would highlight and recognize performance, share a few happy patient stories with each other, and review any new company rollouts.

From time to time, we had other departments like marketing and operations join our call. We were all frustrated with the online attacks. Here we were trying to help patients look and feel great through a much more affordable alternative to the traditional facelift, and the Internet was killing us. We would have meetings and training on how to combat the competitors saying our doctors weren't qualified or it's not a real procedure. You name it; we heard it. And so, in coming up with ideas, in that split moment, the words came over the phone line to the entire field team, which followed with an email just to put a little more salt on it.

"Put your wig and skirt on Ladies and tell them about the great experience you had."

Oh No... No. No. No. No. no! We're not doing that. I didn't do that, and neither did most of the employees. We knew that wasn't the best way. I fielded and made probably 100 calls over the next few days letting consultants know that they did not, nor should, write any reviews online. We could ask patients to write reviews and help improve our online reputation that way. Too late, damage was done, and so a new word was came into our vocabulary.

Astro what? The company behind the Lifestyle Lift was fined $300,000 for "cynical, manipulative, and illegal" activities in the state of New York. Engaging in a practice called "astroturfing," employees of the company were posing as satisfied patients online.[6]

[6] Leiser, Mark; AstroTurfing, 'CyberTurfing' and other online persuasion campaigns; European Journal of Law and Technology; Nov. 1, 2016

This was a big deal for everyone. I can tell you again from working there that it wasn't done with ill intent. It was out of concern to fight the company's reputation. What it was a very bad decision, and sadly, after all these years, people continue to write fake reviews or hide behind the computer saying anything they want, good or bad. We have no way of really knowing what is false and what is true. You can't weigh heavily on anything you read on the Internet. Competition for patients can be intense, especially in areas where there is a plastic surgeon on every corner. Some unscrupulous providers are not above cheating a bit to bring patients in the door. There are many places that offer free services to you if you write a review—they just haven't been caught. I'm not a techie person, but I do know that some of the online doctor review sites can push down or pull forward good and bad reviews. Advertising pays for a lot of what's promoted, so what I would tell you the consumer is to do your own research. Here are a few simple things you can do.

- Check a surgeon's credentials.
- Check to verify Board Certification and Medical License
- Look at before and after photos of their actual patients.
- Ask how long the staff has been there. That tells you a lot
- Ask to speak with previous patients to get their take on the surgeon, his or her staff, and the procedure.
- If you need to, don't be afraid to take time to make your decision.

Now let me expound on that last bullet since I'm from a sales background. I'm not afraid to say I'm in sales, and I train others on how to improve their selling. I don't know why so many people, especially doctors, shy away from it. I'm pretty sure the person who walks in the door knows that if you are a candidate and have the means to afford it, we are going to get you scheduled. So, if you were a patient in front of me, and you want the procedures or services we offer, I am going to try and sell you. I have no problem giving you a few days to make a decision if that's what you really truly need to be comfortable. However, what I'm not comfortable doing is having you share your entire personal story and then pacify you that it's ok to keep thinking.

My job, if you meet the criteria, is to push you out of your comfort zone. I'm here to tell you the truth and help you grow. That's what a great salesperson does. If you want to sit around and think about it for weeks or months, don't bother coming in—seriously. That's like saying I want to lose weight while eating a candy bar.

Lastly, I'll say this. If a doctor, or Patient Coordinator, or anyone on the practice team is bothered by your requests, or you don't feel comfortable with the answers they provided you, find someone else. The ones who are confident in what they do and qualified to do it will willingly share whatever necessary to make you feel comfortable with your decision.

CHAPTER 13: THE DOCTORS

When you work in plastic surgery, you get to work closely with doctors. I've always had such a high level of respect for their years of schooling and superior academics. This respect is because I was always told in school how smart I was if I would just learn to apply myself. What does that even mean? I was a B student with a few sprinkled A's and C's in there; maybe a D if I was really checked out, but I always managed to squeak by and have fun doing it. I was involved in everything from music to sports, even through college. In my own humble brag, I became a pretty well-rounded person. I'm not going to be helping the kids with math homework anytime soon, but I'm ok with that.

Now I mention this because so many of these wonderful doctors, even with their high-level critical thinking, sometimes miss the mark on common sense and the every day what's normal to the average Jane. That's where the Patient Coordinator comes in. I can't tell you how many times I've been asked, "Why do I need a Patient Coordinator?" Really? One word: Connection. Patients need someone to connect with. Docs may not know how or may not have time. There are many reasons they don't teach the people skills needed to interact at a high level in medical school.

I'm not a doctor. I don't know all the science and intricacies of anatomy. I don't diagnose, or recommend, or perform procedures. I leave that up to the experts. What I do know is people. I've coached many doctors in their bedside manner and communication skills over the years. It's like comparing a personal trainer to a physical therapist, two different positions, both potentially needed.

Here I was, sitting down with a surgeon talking to them about where they needed to improve. I look back and think, wow, I really went there. No fear. I had tunnel vision on helping everyone provide the patient with a great experience, so I always looked through the lens of the patient. I've had doctors reach out to me years later, or some I'm still friends with, thank me. We all have something we can learn. Whether you have a Medical Degree or a Masters in the school of Life, we can all do better, learn from others, and keep growing.

I've worked with some truly amazing docs and some real characters. These are a few stories of docs I helped connect with their patients along the way.

Scrubs & Stains

It's Monday morning with a busy schedule. We've lost a few patients on our surgery schedule due to medical clearances. As a consultant, your job is to fill the schedule. I'm meeting with a lovely woman in her late 50's. We've come to the portion of the consultation where we'll be introducing her to our highly talented doctor. When I exit the room to let the doctor know I have a patient for him to meet, the practice manager advises me he is running behind, and she will advise him we are in room three. I make my way back in and spend more time chatting. I have the patient sitting in a chair next to a floor standing mirror when the doctor knocks on the door and enters the room. He smiles politely and walks over to shake her hand. As he makes his way to the patient, I notice his green hospital scrubs are next level wrinkled. I mean rolled-up-in-a-twisted ball-for-a-day wrinkled. I debate on making a lighthearted joke as I normally would when I see something that the patient may raise an eyebrow too, however, decide to refrain in this case.

Dr. X shakes Donna's hand and smiles. "I'm Dr. X. I understand you are interested in facial rejuvenation?"

Donna replies, "Yes. Michelle and I have been discussing which procedure may be right for me."

Dr. X proceeds to go into some brief questioning and has Donna look in the mirror to show her what he can do. While this could be a basic story, I'm about to get to the part where both Donna and I are making bunny faces. You know the face, squished up noses, wide eyes, and pursed lips. The old saying goes, 'you can't smell yourself.' Well, I don't know how this could be possible because the smell was enough to knock over an elephant. Dr. X finished his consultation, and polite thank yous exchanged. When the door shut, Donna and I locked eyes and made faces that had us both immediately burst into laughter.

Dr. X, who is a tremendous surgeon, by the way, had obviously left his scrubs in the washing machine for quite some time before sticking them in the dryer. If you've ever waited too long to dry clothes, you know that the smell of mildew sets in, and it carries an odor that is less than fresh. Young Dr. X lived in a bachelor pad and skipped the laundry lessons in med school. Donna, being a mother, understood, and I explained that while Dr. X is a phenomenal surgeon, the office staff has to help him from time to time with basic life skills.

After Donna left, I sat down with the doc. "Let me ask you a question; you are highly intelligent. I'm guessing your SAT scores were double mine. Did you look in the mirror this morning?"

"Yes. Why?"

"Follow me."

We walked into a consultation room.

"Stand here. Tell me what you see when you look at yourself. Seriously look."

He looked at me and said, "Wrinkled. And... messy."

I said, "Yes, and one more thing."

He looked at me and said, "Sloppy?

"Stinky. Doc, we all love you. You're a great surgeon, but you're wearing clothes that are wrinkled and smell like mildew. If you were a patient meeting a doctor who was wearing wrinkled clothes, smelly like a dead rat, what would you think of them?"

He put his head down. When he looked up, I smiled. "It's the total package doc. You want someone to invest in themselves, but they are investing in you too, and you have to give them the best version of you." This was 15 years ago. To this day, Dr. X wears a suit and tie in every consultation.

The Close Talker

Okay, ladies, and of course, gentleman, if you happen to be reading this. We all know them. *That* person who gets up in your personal space. Who doesn't get that if I can feel your breath on me, you're too close? Seriously, back up. What made it worse was this particular doctor was friendly. When I say friendly, I mean hanging around a little too long in the office, asking unrelated questions, and asking you to come into the office to explain things completely unrelated to the job. Just because you're a doctor doesn't mean the ladies want to date you. And let's be clear, we don't want you in our personal space. Don't flirt with us, it's not cute, and it's unprofessional.

So, it's being done with staff. I've been told it was addressed twice, and now it's bleeding into patients. I'm noticing we have fewer patients than normal scheduling, so as I would always do, I called up the Consultant.

"What's happening?"

"Well, he is scaring patient off. He gets so close to their face, and it's creeping out the patients."

Not good. Off I go. I make it in about 30 minutes to the office. Barely have time to drop my laptop bag when here he comes.

"Michelle, you got a minute?"

"Sure, Doc."

"I want to talk about the Before and After Photos. There's a specific way they need to be taken, let me show you how I want them."

At this point, I'm standing in the exam room, listening as he shows me the blue backdrop. He comes closer; I back up. He leans in again.

See these photos here? These are great before and after photos. Aren't these better?"

"Yes, doc, they are, and we will set up floor markers right away based on the angles we need patients to stand. Can we speak in your office for a minute, please? Here's what I want to say, thank you for always identifying areas we can improve.

I agree we need to have a protocol for taking before and after's and having markers, is a fantastic idea. I'll make sure I communicate that to our medical team at corporate, and we can roll that out in every office. Here's what else I want to talk about."

"What's great about you is that you are so comfortable with the team and the patients. And at the same time, what's important to understand is that what's considered comfortable to one isn't always comfortable to others. I'm going to be blunt—you're making people uncomfortable by not giving them enough personal distance when you communicate. Here let me show you. You stand here."

I moved back a few steps and start talking; he moves up. "No, you stay right where you are." I back up again and put my arms out like a sleepwalker. This is the distance we need you to keep when having a conversation. I put my arms down and take two steps forward, standing way to close for my comfort, but needing to make a point.

"This is not appropriate unless it's your wife, child, dog, cat whatever. Not a patient and not an employee. Ever. Can you see how this would make someone uncomfortable?"

"I guess. I didn't think it was that bad."

"It is, and it is bothering the team and some of our patients. We know you're a great doctor, and we also know sometimes we need help pointing out areas that we may not notice are affecting our communication or are jobs. Just like the before and after photos, right? There's a better way to take them. There's a better way to communicate by giving people a certain amount of distance when you speak to them. I know the last thing you want to do is make a patient feel uncomfortable, so going forward, plenty of distance."

"Ok. You got it."

"You promise?"

"Yes."

"You're not going to eat onions for lunch and try and to come talk to me, are you?"

"LOL, maybe."

He reverted to his old behavior from time to time, but the team knew to step back, and he got it.

The Dumpster Diver

"Come on, Doc, seriously? I can't hide my facial expressions."

"I've been told never to play poker. We can order you some lunch, Doctor B."

"No, No. This is fine. It's still sitting here in the box."

I look at the surgical tech sitting next to me in the break room. We both give the, 'No he didn't look' to each other. The doctor puts the sandwich in one hand, runs his fingers through his hair, shoves the sandwich in his mouth, and flies out the door. "Did he really get that out of the garbage can?"

"Yes, he did!"

I'm visiting this office today and took a break to meet with some of the team individually.

"Has he done this before?"

“All the time.”

I’m in a Seinfeld episode once again. I try talking to him, but he’s always distracted. I wait until the end of the day.

“Doc, you got a minute?”

“Sure, what’s up?”

“Earlier in the break room.” He was still looking at a chart. I cleared my throat and waited until he looked up. “Earlier in the break room, you took food out of the garbage.”

“Did I?”

“Ya did. Now we would be happy to order you lunch and put it in the fridge for you but going into the garbage. Well, I don’t have to tell you all the reasons that’s bad, right?”

“Well, it was just sitting there still in the container.”

“It doesn’t matter. You are a leader in this practice. What type of perception are you giving off to the team when they see you fly into the room like Kramer from Seinfeld? Then push a little garbage around and open a Styrofoam container to eat a half-eaten sandwich? It's nasty, and I know your mama taught you better than that!"

Doc laughed, "Yeah, I got ya."

"OK, no more eating from the garbage can, you come to us when you want us to order you lunch, deal?"

"Deal."

Mr. Jibberish

"He's so awkward. It's uncomfortable in the room with him. He talks to the patient like they're one of his medical colleagues."

"Have you tried talking to him one on one?"

"Yes. OMG, he's the worst. We had a team meeting last week, and he just stood there staring at everyone."

"Alright, let's see what going on."

"Hi Dr. S, my name is Michelle. I work with many of the doctors and consultants regarding how we can improve the consultation and patient experience.

Would you mind if I observed you today for a few visits?"

"That would be fine."

After advising the patient I would be sitting in on her visit, I let Dr. S. take the lead. Dr. S. enters the room and remains standing. Oh boy, rule number one, sit down! I stayed quiet as I listened to him explain the procedures for 40 minutes, using every medical term known to man. I tried to stay engaged, nodding along and smiling, forcing myself not to nod off 10 minutes in. The patient had a blank stare and was trying to be polite, pretending to be engaged.

He talked about his elite schooling and covered every risk one by one. I could see the body language and facial expressions change as the woman seated was wondering when this was going to be over. Dr. S. completed his part of the consultation, shook the patient's hand, and out the door we went.

"How did you think that went?"

"Good."

"No, it did not."

He looked at me, puzzled. “We can’t understand what you’re saying? Look doc, you are uber-smart and no question talented, but when you talk to patients, you gotta speak appropriately to non-medical people. We didn’t go to medical school. Second, you’re scaring everybody off! Of course, we want patients to know the risks, but you just spent 20 minutes covering all the reasons not to do it. Did you ever watch Charlie Brown as I child?”

“Yes. Ok, you’re the teacher.”

“Oh no, really?”

“Yes.”

Dr. S. laughed. “That’s not good.”

“It’s not, but so easy to change. Let’s role-play a few times. I’m the patient, talk to me like you would a patient.” The first go-around, I stopped. “Ok, I’m not six years old starting kindergarten. Now you’re taking it to a new level.”

“Oh, sorry.”

It’s ok. Think about when you went on a first date, how did that go?”

“My wife is a doctor too.”

"LOL, of course, she is. I'm sure she's lovely. Do you have non-physician friends?"

"Yes."

"OK, and do you have hobbies outside of medicine?"

"Yes, I like music."

"What kind of Music?"

"Rap music."

"What? OK. Now Dr. S., with a little flavor! Who's your favorite rapper?"

"Jay Z."

"Ok. Let's try this." We put some music on. "When you listen to music, do you feel more relaxed?"

"Yes."

"OK, start by smiling and asking me a few questions. You don't need to tell me your background; the consultant already covered that. You sound like you have a big ego, and it comes off obnoxious." I smiled. "I say it with love, Doc." He laughed. "Also, cliff notes on the risks. Unless the patient asks for a dissertation on all the awful things that can happen to them, stop giving one. There are risks in everything we do. It's ok to say that. Mention the biggest risks and hopefully why those don't apply to them based their medical history, and our accredited facility, and skills of the surgical team. Is he/she a good candidate, any major medical issues? What the procedures entail, and you're in great hands. Simple, right?"

"Yes."

"Ok, let's try again."

We roll played consultations over three days. Dr. S. had that consultation down, and the patients loved him. He's a very successful plastic surgeon now. He remembers me, and when I hear Jay Z, I always laugh to myself... Bounce with me, Bounce with me.

CHAPTER 14 Don't Sweat The Technique

Do you work on commission? I love that question. I don't get it often, but when I do, I respond with, "Should I? What other profession can you ask someone how they are paid?"

I didn't realize that there were names for it. I had always sold based on my level of knowledge and skill. It wasn't until I started becoming aware of the importance of furthering my education on the profession of sales and management/leadership. If you're in sales, you've likely read books from Zig Ziglar, Brian Tracy, or books like *'Spin Selling'*[7] or *'The Little Red Book of Selling'*[8]. Maybe you've read Dale

---

[7] Spin Selling; Situation. Problem. Implication. Need-Payoff: **By** Neil Rackham

[8] Little Red Book of Selling: 12.5 Principles of Sales Greatness by Jeffrey Gitomer

Carnegie's *'How to Win Friends and Influence People'* or Steven Coveys *'7 Habits of Highly Effective People'*. I loved all of them. It all sounded like what I was doing, but it was reinforcement, and I would always pick up something. Reading keeps you sharp—mentally in the game. I don't care what profession you're in, if you don't keep practicing; you'll lose that skill. Stay sharp. Some of the old school stuff to me feels outdated—the Benjamin Franklin close or the puppy dog close. Yes, these are real techniques; look them up!

I remember this sales manager who fancied asking me if I used this one particular closing technique at a conference.

I asked, "Which one is that?"

She said, "It's when you sit side by side next to the person and present pricing to them."

I smiled. "Well, that sounds great. I do a Michelle close. That's when I make a genuine connection with the person I'm talking to and sit wherever we're both comfortable to discuss the quote."

I'm not against technique at all. I think they're great. I just always want to coach people to do what feels right. Zig Ziglar came up with these techniques in the 1970s. People's buying styles have changed. People are much savvier, and they want to speak with someone who's transparent. No games. Real talk.

I was introduced to NLP[9] in 2010. I remember the company hiring some outside consultants, and my boss at the time asked me if I knew what it was. I said, "Never heard of it." "

Do the research, Michelle." She was always giving me assignments and spoke in riddles. It was like she always wanted me to figure things out myself. It drove me crazy, but she was an awesome boss. I used to get so frustrated when I saw what I believed to be bad decisions being

---

[9] Neuro-linguistic programming is a pseudoscientific approach to communication, personal development, and psychotherapy created by Richard Bandler and John Grinder in California, United States in the 1970s.

made for the company. She would always say, "You hold the power. What does that mean? Years later, I realized I did hold the power; it just took me a while to figure that out.

NLP. Why do I need to know this? It's a psychological approach to implement strategies to sell. It provides lots of tactics to produce a high level of influence. The best way I can describe it is that it's similar to sales psychology. Now that definition could be totally wrong, so if you're an NLP guru, apologies. When I was introduced to the book *'The Psychology of Persuasion and Influence'* by Robert Cialdini, Ph.D., I was intrigued. In his book, he talks about the six principles of persuasion and how these strategies work at a cognitive level. It helps people understand how the brain works and what behaviors can be created using principles that motivate someone to act. The principles are:

> Reciprocity
> Scarcity
> Authority
> Consistency

> Liking

> Consensus

I've read that book at least twenty times. It's highlighted and torn up, but its foundation made complete sense to me. Sales are all about psychology, and I had no idea what I was already doing had real techniques behind it.

CHAPTER 15: You Better Recognize

2011, "So, let me get this straight. I've spent the last five years building a department, traveling all over the country, hiring, training, and coaching salespeople, building a team that's doing very well I might add. Now you want to bring in someone at a higher level because they have more years of experience and look better on paper? Does the doctor know about this?"

"He looks good on paper to investors, blah, blah blah." *Don't cry, Michelle, hold it together.*

I was angry, sad, and every emotion in between. How could they let someone come in and take over? I don't understand? It was explained to me that they needed someone who lived in the corporate office city, and they knew I wouldn't move to Michigan. This would be a moot point these days, but technology wasn't as up to date in the virtual world. Still, it was wrong, and everyone knew it.

I'm sure Dr. Kent was getting pushback from a few senior team members. I can imagine how many conversations took place that went something like, "Look David, we really need to get someone to oversee sales who can take us to the next level. I know you think Michelle is great, but this person would be her mentor. Someone with experience working with fortune 500 and 100 companies, plus we need someone here every day. The company has tripled in size. It's time. Don't worry; we will take care of Michelle."

They also wanted someone who had an MBA. I wonder how long they sat around figuring out how they could justify screwing me over. I was pacified by receiving the first-ever and made up, "Lifestyle Lift Merit Award."

"You choose an online school, Michelle and, we will pay for your MBA classes."

Now maybe to some that doesn't sound like a bad deal, and understand, I was and am still grateful. What was bothersome was that I knew it was to appease me. It was the consolation prize and the everyone-gets-a-trophy. I wanted to scream and throw mine in the garbage. What happened to earning the win? Looking back, I did win. I started my online MBA classes the following month.

What makes this story so comical is that the gentleman they hired for the position not only did not have a master's degree, he never moved to corporate.

Ok, this is harder than I thought. Come on, how do you go from first place to second gracefully? Who wants to take direction from someone who knows nothing about the business? I don't care what degrees of experience you have—if you haven't done the job, how are you truly going to lead others? There's probably 1% of people out there who could be effective in doing that. I'm not saying it can't happen. I know there are some successful coaches out there who haven't played, but in this case, we're talking about predominately female team members and predominately female patients.

Whenever a new person came on board with the company, especially men, they would have this glossed over fascination with the business. It would take months to grasp how this business model worked. We weren't retail and were different than a standard medical practice. This was unchartered territory unless you came from the inside. Even now, people who work for this type of business model, who are hired from the outside, struggle. It's a category all its own.

I seriously prayed about it and went through all the pros and cons. I was hurt—more like crushed. My heart was starting to turn stone cold, and I was trying to fight it every day. I'm not going to let them steal my joy. I kept telling myself, "I'm not going to let them change my feelings," but deep down, it was literally and figuratively eating me alive. I wasn't sure if I was more upset about the job or that I was eating my feelings and getting fat!

Thankfully, I was given an opportunity to keep my distance and work on special projects. My team and I spent the next four months building a program that would be monumental to this business model.

We were asked to work with an outside consultant team to develop concepts to better influence buyers... walk us through everything. "We want to understand how you do it, what you say and why you say it. You and your team—what makes you the best in the industry." And so, for the next four months, we documented every word, every phrase, every concept and technique, and incorporated it into designing a program that combined personality profiling concepts, to this day, has a huge influence on sales training inside the aesthetic industry.

Looking back, I don't know if I would have brain-dumped everything exactly this way. However, it worked out for everyone, and I look at it as having an incredible impact even if it doesn't have my signature attached.

Between our locked-door whiteboard meetings, I kept limited interaction with my new boss. I was happy to have a separate project to work on, and I'm pretty sure everyone knew best to leave me alone. They knew I was salty, but oh well. If they cared, they wouldn't have done it, so it wasn't my problem. I kept justifying to myself that I had a job, I was making a difference, and quite frankly, I was making a pretty great paycheck. Plus, I figured it was only a matter of time more changes and employee turnovers occurred again. *Patience Michelle, patience.*

When I did have meetings, I would hold back my, "I really want to punch someone in the face," especially when I would hear things like, "Now Michelle, this is a teachable moment." Oh really, is it? I would smile through my teeth and painfully watch the second hand move until our time was up. Meetings were set up on the half-hour, so I would pass my team members in the hallway and high five as we walked by each other. Keep your head up.

My colleague, who I had hired and had been my right hand for years, was hiding a secret. She was expecting! Having been in the health and fitness industry for years, she was in phenomenal shape and didn't show until she was about six months. Even then, she could have passed for eating a little too much from a weekend bender. This was the exact opposite of my pregnancy experience, where I looked like a balloon ready to pop—at 6 months. With all the management changes, we kept it quiet because it was like Hunger Games—survival of the fittest.

There was a constant stream of changes. People were getting promoted/demoted, hired, and fired. New people were coming in droves. There was a department for a department. What was once a coveted work hard to hold a senior-level position was becoming a dime-a-dozen. I was told after I left the company it was worse. If an idea came up, the next thing you know, a new department would pop up, and an outside consultant was hired. And when that happened, you would be stuck spending your time walking them through the business instead of on driving the business forward.

Toward the end, I flat out refused. *Nope, I'm not doing it.* Why when we have so many capable people who work here that can help us? New ideas; different experiences. OK, I get that; however, some leaders were notorious for putting up a job description just to placate others. They had no intention of internally filling the position. What was worse, I can't be completely certain, but it was pretty obvious people getting positions who weren't the best fit because they were playing the game or cozying up to the right person.

I've learned over the years, high-ups bring in their own people. It's not about whose qualified; it's about who you know. My advice to young people looking for a job is to start networking as much as you can because nine times out of ten, it's who you know.

I remember one gentleman being hired for a pretty high-paying, senior position because he was a buddy with another member. He was allegedly losing his home and needed a job. He made a phone call and there you go, no experience, no consideration of an internal candidate—just part of the boy's club, come on in let's roll out the red carpet.

After my partner announced her pregnancy to HR and the management team, we strategized how her travel would look. Her husband was in the military and was transferred to a city that was not close to a nearby airport where we had a location. Unfortunately, at this point, she was no longer directly reporting to me, so we knew that it would be more complicated. It eventually led to her end of employment.

Now, let me say, not only was she my right hand, she was a great employee; one of the best and the brightest. She was the employee that every company needs and the person that exudes positivity. If my heart wasn't already bruised, I had to watch the person who had become like a sister ultimately be pushed out—different dynamics, different expectations. Her schedule was changing, and theirs provided more demands. I told myself that when we own our own company, we would work around a mom's schedule (and now we do).

There is so much talent out there, and not enough companies accommodate for this. It wasn't always like this, but with the new regime, the boys' club ruled. You could be on the bus or not. If you were on the bus or played nice in the sandbox, you would likely be safe. If not, you were a problem and would be pushed out one way or the other.

It felt like our family was crumbling.

One team member, who worked in a director role, became a target when he approached some colleagues and boss after identifying numbers that appeared manipulated to present to Dr. Kent so that new programs would be approved. When the Director brought up the inaccuracy of the reports, he was told it would be addressed. Another senior member later found out and said to the whistleblower, "You've got a bull's-eye on your back. You need to get on the same page with us, or you won't have a job by the end of the month. We have to get things approved, so don't worry about the numbers."

The Director resigned from his position thirty days later and took a job as a VP at another company. Another great employee and colleague was hired and fired twice because she spoke up on issues that weren't being addressed in the field. I asked her if she was a glutton for punishment and that they needed to institute a double jeopardy rule for business! For me, it became quite common for me to be told not to speak to Dr. Kent.

"Don't speak to David."

"Really, what would you like me to do when he calls and asks me to tell him what's going on, lie?" I'm not going to do that."

We don't lie in our family, but this wasn't family anymore, this was business, and it was getting dirty.

One of my last days at the job, I had flown in for a meeting. I remember sitting in the boardroom with some of my fellow field directors. I had stepped out of sales at this point and moved over to operations. I knew that was the only way I could stay on with the company and not be bitter. None of us had any idea why we were there. One by one, we were called into a room that had a chair set up in the middle and a team of corporate managers, HR, and senior business team members.

This is a true story; I'm not kidding. I still think about how odd and demeaning this was, and how this would never have happened in the earlier years. We had now become, in my view, a company of distrust. Once trust is gone, it's only a matter of time.

I shook my head, "Is this for real? You want me to sit in that hot seat? Is there a bright light to flash in my eyes as well?"

One of my colleagues lost it after what he called an hour of hell. He resigned soon after, as well. I always noticed that when someone resigned, it was considered a good thing. It doesn't matter what company you work for—when you leave... everything that was wrong is your fault.

I took a seat, and they began a line of questions.

"Michelle, we need to know if we have the right people in place before we go into the New Year. We want you to go down the list of each office manager and determine what changes need to be taken."

My response was one of shock. "Like this? Okay, why are some of these people who have no relationship with the offices in here?"

"Well, they all have some interactions with the offices."

"Yes, but that's a lot of subjective input, don't you think?"

"We want to take everything into consideration."

"Whatever, let's get started."

I was running operations at the time for seven locations, responsible for a 35 million dollar a year region. The questions pertained mainly to the leadership in each office, and on whether I believed we had the right people leading the teams. I'm sure this was someone's brilliant idea, and everyone at the time thought it was great, but where they missed the mark was any consideration for the leader.

It felt more like being on the chopping block because we were getting rapid-fire questions coming from every department—no warning, no preparation. One person surrounded by a team of people in a large room with a dozen banquet chairs circled around. Maybe they were going for intimate setting. Nah, more like intimidating.

I remember Dr. Kent popping through the grey double doors, taking a seat in the back on the windowsill. We locked eyes. I forgot where I was for a moment and wondered if he was thinking, "What in the world is going on in here? What are we doing" That's what I was thinking.

"What would you say about Donna?"

"She's a great manager."

"What makes you say that?"

"Well, she creates a team environment and communicates all policies and procedures (we rolled out new policies and procedures practically every week). She is tenured, and follows up with patients in a timely manner. The office has seen year over year growth, and low turnover."

"What do you think about her communication style and how she speaks?"

"How she speaks?"

"Yes, it can come off, well...hard to understand, a bit jumbled, and sometimes it comes off... well... not as polished."

What I wanted to say is, "Maybe you guys need some diversity training." I responded with, "Nope, don't experience that."

He didn't come out and say it, but I knew what he was saying, and so did everyone in the room.

"Donna has been with us for years. If she communicates in a way that may be different than what some of you are used to, then we can work with her on that. However, she is doing a great job and has been a loyal employee. It's not easy to manage these offices and doctors and patients. I believe she and all the managers in my region are doing a great job. Are they without issues? Are any of us?"

"We have the number one producing region in the company because we are a team. We stay focused on our goals, we support each other, we communicate, we have fun, and we are DIVERSE. I'm happy with everyone, and if there is someone I believe as the head of this team, which I understand I am responsible for, I will be sure to communicate to the appropriate person on coaching up or coaching out, so I am comfortable with all my managers" I stood up. "Are we all set?"

When I resigned, I was offered my job back this time with the title to go with it. I would be their VP of Sales. The gentleman they had hired to fill my shoes, as expected, made his way out. Dr. Kent pleaded with me not to leave. He knew the connection I had with the field, the results, and the work ethic I brought to my job. He asked me to take a week off to decide and didn't want me to make a rash decision.

I shut down my laptop for the first time in years. It felt weird, but I needed to make sure I was certain. I made the decision to take a trip back to corporate. I couldn't say I was 100 percent. I'm sitting at dinner with everyone, laughing and telling stories. We had some great people, but the underlying feeling was that the direction and leadership in place wasn't my style. Do I want to keep playing this game, or do I want to hold my head high and walk away at the height of winning? One of the outside consultants said to me, "When you moved into operations, the team thought you were just sales and were all expecting you to fail; fall on your face. You really showed them and hit it out of the park!"

This statement sat with me, all night the night before my final decision. Let me play that back… "The 'team' thought you would fall on your face." What kind of people in leadership positions say this? I knew it wasn't coming from Dr. Kent. I knew he didn't believe that, but he wasn't running the day-to-day. Why would anyone want to work with someone that didn't believe in them? You want me to fail?

Some say business isn't personal; I disagree. So when I was brought into the room for what was expected to be me accepting the position, I was asked what I thought leadership was. I responded with, "I know what it isn't."

I declined the position and I left on my terms with my head held high.

CHAPTER 16: Blessings

2012 I took a short stint as head of operations for a multiple location aesthetics company that was struggling. Through that job, I made a friend for life—a crazy Jewish woman from New York with a larger than life personality. She is the hardest working person I know and has a heart of gold. We were kindred spirits. She introduced me to her old boss, who wanted to start a plastic surgery company.

It was an exciting opportunity that ignited my passion. We opened 5 locations together travelling across the country. We hired team members, scouted locations, purchased equipment, furniture, created marketing materials and policies. We were Human Resources, Financing, Operations, Marketing and Sales. The only thing we didn't do were the surgeries but quite honestly after you've watched enough, you start to think maybe that's not too difficult! (I'm completely kidding, cheers to the amazing docs that go to school for years for their skills)

It was ground up, fourteen-hour days and while we had a decent run, the cost of marketing was absurd, and we ended up dissolving the business. Starting a company is a tremendous learning experience. No matter how much you think you know, there is no guarantee. You have to learn from every experience. They say fifty percent of all new business fail. You've got a twenty five percent chance to last even a year. We lasted two.

The good news was that we followed each other to our next startup venture. I went first out on my own, going into different private practice plastic surgery practices, helping streamline their business. I would sit in on every pre-op and watch surgeries as much as possible. There were so many different reasons people came in. I loved observing how different the doctor's techniques were and style of leadership inside their practice.

The freedom on my schedule was amazing. I had wrapped myself up so much in work that I hadn't had time for myself. In my entire six years at Lifestyle Lift, I took one vacation. It was my wedding, and I took five days. How stupid is that? If you're reading this and have a job, take your days—all of them! My identity was work. I needed to get some hobbies and do something non-work related. When an opportunity came up to travel to Europe, I jumped on it. Within a month or so from returning from my trip, I was blessed with the biggest job of my life. I was going to become a mom.

So... I want to know who's having it all? Who are these women? Nobody I know. It's stressful, and I only have one child! Seriously, someone wrote a book about how *you can have it all*—lady, please. I'm exhausted, and I was once running circles around people. Now, I can barely spell circle! My number one job is mom, and I am going to figure this out.

Then I met the world's coolest boss. She was tough. Ooh, she was tough, and she had a gigantic heart. If she liked you, she loved you, and if she didn't, well, you better get out of her way. We called her the Black Widow. She spoke six languages and dripped in Chanel. She had a way with doctors like I had never seen before. She knew how to use both brains and beauty in a way that commanded respect. Sometimes I would just sit back and observe her movement; her body language and her style of communication. Her influencing skills were remarkable. Her keen ability to sniff out bullshit was amazing. She would eat you for breakfast and put you right in your place—mostly men—and I loved every minute of it. She scared a lot of people, but not me. I loved having a strong female alpha boss. She saw my value and elevated me as a great leader does with their team. She also respected my time, something I had never experienced. What would take some people three days would take me three hours. She worked hard and played harder. Everything was first class.

Who gets a call from a boss who says, "It's been a long month, you've all worked hard, we're flying to Greece for a few days on me." True story. I loved the team. We didn't have the ideal investors, but the plastic surgeons, team members, and patients were amazing. I worked remote, traveled for big events, and practice acquisitions. We built it from scratch, and I loved, loved, loved my colleagues. These were some of the best years of my career.

CHAPTER 17: Know Before You Go

2015 I took a great part-time consulting job in plastic surgery. "What do you do for work, Michelle?" "Me, I look at naked bodies for a living." That's right, young and old short, tall, large, big, and small. You name it, and I've seen it all (Yes, I write rhymes). It's interesting to me what some people find bothersome, and other areas that they could care less about. As a consultant or coach, you have to be careful not to tell someone what you believe they need to change.

1. You are not a doctor, and 2. It's all about what they see in the mirror.

Here's what's interesting. Most people are so self-conscious about their appearance. I can tell you there's no reason to be. There's nothing weird about the way you look, and there's nothing to be afraid of.

Cosmetic enhancements have come a long way since I started. Great results can come from both surgical and non-surgical options. I've seen great outcomes from procedures that offer more subtle enhancements

Here are some basic things to know:

Experience Matters

Medical Spa laws regarding a physician's supervision requirements differ state to state. Regarding the practice of aesthetics, in many states, Nurse Practitioners can open their own practice. Some states require onsite physicians, and others require a physician oversight. The important take away is that a medical professional should always perform all medical treatments. You want to make sure the facility has proper licensing to meet state regulations. Always do your research on experience, training, and legal requirements. Only well-trained, experienced professionals should perform Non-surgical Procedures. I've seen injectors receive minimal training with practice on an orange then be asked to inject on real people. Yes, our bright, beautiful Florida orange, not foreheads.

I remember one day a nurse had come back from a one-day training on injecting. A patient came in wanting Botox. The consultant was excited to get a scheduled patient while the Injector looked at us with fear in her eyes. "No way, I'm not ready." The consultant responded with, "We need this sale." As the boss, I made the decision to let the patient walk. Can you imagine if this person had injected that woman? With only one day of practice on an orange? No oversight, just a young woman with a needle. Yeah, that's reality, and that why you need to get all the facts.

I get asked, "Do you know anyone who's died from plastic surgery?" Sadly, yes. Complications? Infection? Yes. It's the worst thing imaginable. You don't hear about this, but we, as insiders know it. Settlements and signed nondisclosures prevent them from talking about it.

As a potential patient, you have to get the facts, and as we say at MyCoachMD, know before you go. This is one of the reasons people come to us. We have done the vetting for you, and will only put you in front of doctors with the right credentials. You are still the people who ultimately make the decision on who will perform your procedure. We will steer you in the direction that meets the criteria for experience.

Unfortunately, today, there is no requirement that a physician who's actually trained in the discipline perform cosmetic surgery. In fact, cosmetic procedures are not just offered by board-certified plastic surgeons, but by physicians of every background, including family physicians, dermatologists, gynecologists, ophthalmologists, and oral surgeons—really any physician initially trained in other fields. Here's my caveat to that, non-surgical and surgical are two very different options. I know plenty of great doctors who are not plastics offering non-surgical treatments, with the proper training. However, when it comes to surgery, in my opinion, there's no grey area. If you have a aesthetic surgery, I recommend you go to a Board-Certified Plastic Surgeon who has formal specialized training, experience, skill and knows how to handle any critical situation that may arise.

Many doctors promote as Board-certified. You always want to make sure that the certification they are talking about is by the American Society of Plastic Surgeons (ASPS), American Board of Plastic Surgery (ABPS), American Academy of Facial Plastic and Reconstructive Surgery (AAFPRS) or for outside of the United States, International Society of Aesthetic Plastic Surgery (ISAPS).

CHAPTER 18: Lift Off

2009. Good Morning Consultants! Our weekly sales calls were awesome. We called them LIFT Off Calls, and we started with music to get our team pumped up. Our trainer was my right hand and had become my best friend. She was such an integral part of the building of the company. We all adored her. What was great about the team I assembled was that everyone started as a Consultant in the field had tremendous experience and were good people.

I always believe it is difficult to bring someone in from the outside. I worked for a company that hired a sales director from the outside, and she was never able to really get her footing. She was likable, but the respect wasn't there. They tried putting her in to perform consultations, but she wasn't connecting with patients, which only made it worse. Everyone knew she wasn't well suited to the job, and it continued to snowball until eventually she was released.

I don't think companies truly understand the financial impact of hiring the wrong people. You gotta walk the walk and talk the talk. You also need to hire people who can influence and inspire others. There are some people who are suited to playing the field and others who are better coaching from the sidelines or watching from the stands. Companies should look for leaders with a passion for life and business. Really, when it comes down to it on the very basic level, the position of sales consultant, coordinator, coach, whatever you want to call it, is about helping people better themselves.

Our calls were fun and informative. The exact opposite of what conference calls typically are. We would take roll call with shout outs. It was used to pump people up, and everybody felt the energy. It wasn't a sales call; it was about lifting our team up to lift others up. Our patients came to us when they were down, and it was our job to lift them up. We wanted to lift people's spirits. The transformation of the patients was amazing, and those were the special golden nuggets inside Lifestyle Lift.

CHAPTER 19: IT'S BUSINESS

The executive boardroom seats about fourteen. All chairs are filled, and I'm one of three females invited to the table. I arrive early, as usual, and take a seat. I glance over to see a book on the table called '*WHY SHE BUYS.*' For the next two and a half hours, I'm listening to men analyze and question each chapter and their thoughts on excerpts from Bridget Brennan's book.

I'm casually making eye contact with my female counterparts to read their body language. Seriously, is this happening? Are they feeling the same as I am? The comments are getting more ridiculous as it goes on.

Some well-intentioned men were sitting in the room, and I'm by no means a male basher—far from it. I have the greatest men in the world in my life; my husband, father, brother-in-law, uncles, cousins, best friends—all stellar men. I'm talking about the old boys club network that exists in a corporate setting. How is it that a company with almost an all women consumer base has three women representing the demographic?

I was told early on in my career that business was like playing a game of chess. I hate chess. *Play the game... I don't want to play the game.* Truth is, you have to learn to play if you want to win. Once you win, then you can call the shots. OK, game on.

I was living in two different worlds. On days I was in the field, I would be meeting with patients and team members. It was all about the emotion, connection, how people felt, and how I made them feel. When I was sitting with the corporate decision-makers, I had to keep all the emotion out of the room. Stick to the facts, Michelle. Keep it direct. Follow the alpha male playbook. If you show emotion, you're labeled as emotional or hormonal, so keep it cool.

I remember one time being called as a witness to be interviewed in a potential class-action lawsuit. I was told it would be a room full of their lawyers, a videographer, stenographer, and members of our legal team—10 people—all men. Up until now, I had done a few mediations and small case interviews, but never anything like this—hours of questioning. I was defending the company and my integrity. I sat at the end of the long table with a camera in my face and every word being documented. We had an in-house lawyer, who I adored. He attended with me and on breaks, kept reassuring me I was doing well.

During the recorded deposition, I went question-by-question, line-by-line. Hours of questioning and reviewing of every form and document I ever created or had my hands on. Do you remember this? Why did you say it like this? Did you mean to say it this way? The lawyer kept throwing jabs, and I kept blocking. I knew my work. I knew what we were doing was helping people, and I wasn't going to break, no matter how difficult and exhausting.

When the interview—or interrogation, as it felt like—ended, I went back to my hotel room. I sat on the edge of the bed, put my head down, and cried for an hour. The next day, I got a "heard you did well at the deposition, good job." Good Job? I was numb, my face flushed, but smiled through it. *Don't cry, Michelle. Don't you dare cry.*

I hated playing the game. I wanted it to go back to the way it was when we were family. Everyone liked each other. Now it's about spreadsheets and numbers, and how many more surgeries we can add, and maybe we should open retail hours. Wait. What? These are medical practices. In the famous words of The Notorious Biggie Smalls, "Mo Money, Mo Problems."

The recruiting for doctors got quicker, and we were turning over and growing fast. The old were getting pushed out for the new team with new ideas and experience. The problem was, what we had wasn't broken, but it was certainly getting there. Towards the end of my time, meetings and onsite visits were the worst. Everyone was fake. One senior member told me that I was too by-the-book and needed to loosen up. He used to call me by my last name. Come on, Emmick, have a few drinks with me. It's after hours. *Yeah; no.* So, you can justify your sloppy frat-boy behavior? No thanks. Don't get me wrong I like to loosen up and have fun; in the right environment with the right people. Heavily drinking alone with a boss, or with direct reports, not so much.

I recently started networking with a gentleman who has a Rolodex® of private equity investors and Wall Street who's-who's. He mentioned to me how the aesthetic industry is in high demand with investors. He said he was in talks with an aesthetic company that may be purchased.

"Wow, that's exciting."

He followed up with, "Yes, and I'm going to put Mr. X in as the CEO."

Wow, not so exciting. I knew exactly who he was speaking of—a gentleman with a less than stellar reputation both personally and professionally. And once again, another lost opportunity to do something amazing by placing well respected and experienced female leaders at the helm. It's an almost all-female consumer and employee business! For people that have so many degrees and big-time professional experience, they sure miss the things right in front of their faces. We don't need to read a book on why women buy.

CHAPTER 20: Redline

2008 was a tough year. The economy took a turn, and they say it was the most severe financial crisis since the Great Depression. Lifestyle Lift took a setback like all companies, and we all knew cutbacks had to be made. Anywhere we could make adjustments from spending, payroll, etc., was going on behind the scene. We worked hard to keep everyone's spirits in a positive place, so we didn't nosedive like many other businesses.

It was not easy. Our lift off calls went from once a week to daily. We spent almost every week in Michigan. We talked about challenges as a team, and though we lost a few good consultants along the way, most of the team weathered the storm.

It was told to me that while cutbacks were taking place, a few of the executives went through and were redlining employees. I've been told that when my name came up on the list, one of the executives tried to redline mine, and Dr. Kent said, "Never. Michelle, she stays no matter what."

I never forgot that story. There was so much deception and manipulation that went on behind closed doors, and it was crazy. We were a real-life soap opera. They used to say there were two camps. Your fate was determined by whose camp you chose. I watched my colleagues get knocked down like dominos. When you're talking about millions of dollars, power and greed follow. And when money flows, typically, the underlying cause of self-destruction follows.

It felt like everyone was vying for control and wanted a piece of the company. There were constant closed-door gossip sessions and side conversations where employees were the key stakeholders and who would get a piece of the pie when the company sold. There were promises made around every corner. Everyone with an office felt they were entitled to a bite. There were regular "alleged" stories of infidelity, thousands of dollars in payoffs, and luxury, hotels, and flying first class—all on the company dime. It was a hay day with money that wasn't theirs. They were Poppin' bottles and Makin' it rain while us blue-collar folks did the heavy lifting and looked on.

I remember flying in with other senior members to complete an in-office training. Olive Garden had been ordered for the staff. One of the employees asked one of the senior team members if he wanted something to eat.

Without hesitation, he responded with, "No, of course not, we're going to get our dinner at Ruth Chris after the meeting."

I wanted to run. I was so embarrassed. "I love Olive Garden!" I quickly responded.

I thought to myself, "So you get to drink ridiculously expensive bottles of wine and eat filet at an expensive steakhouse while the team eats moderately priced (and still delicious, however) pasta. "Do you not have the emotional intelligence to realize how that comes off? Or is it that you don't care. Why would you? You're thinking you're getting 400million when the company sells."

At the end of the training, I got the usual, "Emmick, you coming?"

"No thank you, I'm just gonna head back to the hotel."

"Come on, come have a drink with us."

I was taking my master's classes online. So, I had an easy out excuse. I said earlier I wasn't good at poker, and I couldn't bring myself to sit there and act phony for two hours. I pulled it off during the day, but by the nighttime, it was much more likely that if I had to deal with them any longer, I could potentially lose it. I stayed behind, helped clean up, and had some good laughs with the office team. Olive Garden was quite tasty, I might add. Breadsticks. Enough said.

Like a bright flashing light, the warning signs were there. I'm not saying money isn't important; it's hugely important, you can't have a business without it. But you also need to know how to manage it, and these fools acted like they had a limitless pool of funds and knew how to spend it.

Why wouldn't they? It wasn't there's to blow.

CHAPTER 21: Show Me the Money

So, here's the deal. Plastic surgery is big business. Last year men and women spent close to 18 billion dollars on cosmetic procedures. Technologies have advanced, and business continues to grow. Women continue to consume around 90% of the market. However, men are becoming much more open to cosmetic procedures, specifically non-surgical options, which are a huge percentage of the market.

There's always the latest and greatest, the newest procedure. The efficacy—that's a word you hear used repeatedly by reps—which is a fancy word for results. What works, what doesn't? It's a marketing game, and the big players win. If you've got thousands of Instagram followers, paid influencers, compensated celebrity endorsers, and a marketing campaign, the chances are that the product will make it to the top.

Practices are sold expensive equipment, sometimes upwards of $250,000. Is it the best product on the market? Maybe, maybe not, but guess which procedure they are going to push? You are correct! They need to pay off that expensive piece of machinery they bought.

“Should I order this?”

“Order what, Mom?”

“This cream I saw on an Infomercial that says it will erase wrinkles.”

“Are you serious mom? You do know that’s marketing, right? Let me guess it had a medical doctor validating its claims? Well, then sure, go buy that bottle of erase away the wrinkles. Let me know how that works for you.”

The number of times I have heard, “I wasted my money; this didn’t work.” Here’s the big take away. Years ago, nobody used heavy marketing; now everybody uses it. Some put ads in the newspaper; some run commercials, some use digital marketing, social media, and direct mailers. There are plastic surgeons and cosmetic surgeons on every corner, and companies are supporting them in their efforts. You can't be successful without marketing. It's all about word of mouth, referrals… how about an Instagram page with thousands of fake followers? Don't get it twisted—you are being sold. Doctors that don't think they are selling, think again, you are in sales too.

I teach people to sell, and I do it ethically. I cover how to be observant, study your body language, and how you communicate that will, in turn, help better communicate with you the consumer in a way that will support your decision to schedule a service or procedure. I teach people this, and I'm okay with that.

I don't think sales are dirty if you do it for the right reasons. I can tell you there are a lot of people out there that don't have your best interest in mind. One of the reasons I started my business was to educate people, to save them from the marketers pushing their product like a mall kiosk employee pushing their samples. Yes, there are people that will look you in the eye and tell you what you want to hear. Show you the greatest before and after pictures, knowing all too well the results won't come close to what you're looking for. It's heartbreaking, and it's true. And it can be a ruthless game.

It's not uncommon that two people wanting the same services or procedures could be sold at a different price. I remember attending a meeting for a company, and the aesthetic reps were talking about their sales process and what makes them successful. One of the women chimed in and said, "I just look at their shoes and handbag, and that's how I determine what to charge."

Did she just say that? Don't get me wrong—there are situations to extend different pricing. Maybe it's a promotion or a same month surgery; there are many reasons but prices based on someone's shoes and handbag? That's not one of them. It doesn't matter what profession you're talking about—there are people with good and bad intentions. While you would think that wouldn't happen in the field of medicine, you're crazy. We're dealing with elective medicine, but even hospitals and large health systems are managed by high paying CEOs. They spend millions on marketing to attract patients. Pharmaceutical companies invest billions of dollars in the development of new drugs and just as much on promoting them. How many times do you see a drug commercial on television?

CHAPTER 22: Keep it Clean

"OMG! I'm so excited. What is it am I getting again?"

Is this lady serious? I walk out of my office.

"I just wanted to come out and introduce myself. Congratulations, what did you decide to have done?"

"Something with my face."

"Which procedure?"

"I'm not sure."

"Let me take a look. Oh, how exciting, you decided to get a facelift."

Stop right there. Why would it ever be ok that a woman getting a facelift doesn't know it? It's not. This is one of the many reasons I bring up education. You may think this is a one of a kind story, but it's not. I'm not shaming my coworkers or trying to make the patient feel bad. I'm trying to explain that if you're deciding to have a procedure, you better know what you're having done.

There are so many options out there. Vastly different price points and different results. Skincare products, just like non-surgical cosmetic procedures, are all different, and some are better for you than others.

I am not a skincare expert—not even close. Embarrassingly, and my esthetician and dermatology friends reading this would be shaking their heads, many nights I don't wash my face before bed, and I use very limited products, a cleanser infrequently, moisturizer and sunscreen. That's it. I don't think I'm alone in this either. I'm overwhelmed with products, and when people start talking to me about the steps—cleanse, scrub, moisturize, serum, toners, exfoliants, and SPF—I mean seriously? Do people do this?

I remember working with a company discussing a rollout of their new skincare line. There were five of us in the room while my colleague presented us with the six products. He went through each product one by one, providing us a full description of all the ingredients. If there was a dialogue bubble over my head, I would have read, “First of all, nobody cares about something we can’t spell or pronounce, just tell us what does this stuff do and why would I need it.”

He finishes his presentation, and everyone smiles and says, “Great job.” Well, sorry to be the Debbie Downer in the room. Our patients aren’t buying that. And as usual, I receive the deer in the headlights, ‘who does this bitch think she is’ look on their faces.

“No woman is going to use six products. People want simple, easy, convenient, affordable, and products that do what they say they are going to do.” I turn to the only other female in the room, who, God bless her, would agree with whoever is speaking. “Jan, would you agree?” She gives a half shrug and says, “Yes.”

I stand up and say, “Give me 5 minutes.” I leave the room and come back with six female colleagues. “Ladies, let me get your opinions. Very simply, what do you think of this skincare product line?”

Every response: "Too many products." I give a stone-cold stare over to the presenter. "Thanks, everyone." I close the door. "I know you put a lot of effort into this line and presentation, but we have to offer something that works for everyday women. Is there a market for six products? Of course. Is it the market for our demographic? I don't believe it is."

A few months went by, and a three-product skincare line was rolled out. I think it did pretty well. I never used it. What I know is that many people want convenience. I do believe that everyone is unique, and you do need to take care of your skin if you want it to look good. Our skin is aging from both intrinsic and extrinsic factors. You can't do much about genetics however, you can improve your skin based on the environment and your lifestyle choices—habits like smoking and drinking, what we eat, activity, stress, hormonal changes, and overall, how we take care of our skin.

A dermatologist is medically trained to give patients treatment for medical skin conditions and skin diseases through prescribing the use of topical creams and oral drugs. A licensed Aesthetician offers non-prescription solutions like skincare products and can help improve the appearance of your skin overall. There are Aestheticians and Estheticians. Both are licensed skincare specialists, and the biggest variance is the type of clients they work with and the setting they work in. Whomever you to choose to see for your skincare needs, verify their experience training, certifications, and licensing.

CHAPTER 23: Under Pressure

I'm comfortable saying I'm in sales. Most people are afraid of the word—doctors especially.

"Ooh... you don't want to tie a medical procedure with sales."

"Why Not? Are you giving it away for free? It's an elective procedure, right? So the person doesn't need to have it, they want to have it?"

Salespeople get a bad rap. It's right up there with going to the dentist. I was in a meeting once and was asked, "Why do you think we have so many people that don't show for their free consultation?"

"Nothing is for free, and they don't want to be sold."

Sales are a part of life. We all sell. Whether it's convincing your friends to go out on Friday night or getting your kids to do their homework.

The high-pressure sales approach. I used to hear that described when people would talk about large national chains in aesthetics. What exactly does that mean? Should I be offended? They are talking about us anyway, and I happen to lead the largest national chain, so let's hear what they are saying about me.

Hard sellers typically use aggressive, physical gestures, including finger-pointing, forceful language, and emotional appeal to convince others to purchase their service or product. Salespeople using soft selling techniques, conversely, use a softer voice to rationally inform customers about their products, and exhibit more courteous mannerisms, such as smiling, giving others a chance to ask questions, and providing information via brochures and pamphlets to give consumers time to digest information.

Hmm... ok, so I should speak softly and give someone some brochures to look at? Whenever someone says to me, "I'm here for information," I respond with, "And then what? Throw the brochure in your junk drawer? Because that's what I do with a brochure." Well, either that or in the garbage. I certainly don't get forceful or point my finger at someone. I'm not locking them in the room to give me their money. Let me keep reading and see what I can find.

Excerpt found on mbaskool.com regarding high-pressure selling

1. **Endless Chatter**: This is one of the shrewdest techniques used by a salesperson during high-pressure selling. Here, the salesperson keeps explaining the benefits of the service or product. The tone used is friendly but persuasive.

I'm a chatty Cathy. I hope the person thinks I'm friendly. I check yes.

2. **Emotional manipulation**:

Salespeople usually rely on emotional manipulation to pressure customers into buying. For example, they will ask a person who wants something to imagine how they would feel and turning him emotional.

Yes, I do that, absolutely! Why wouldn't I? Who doesn't want to visualize how they are going to look and feel? I do that for myself in my sleep and pretty much throughout the day. I'm all about visualization, and I'm pretty sure most women are. I'm visualizing the hot fudge Sundae I want to eat later. Check yes again; this statement is True!

3. **Limited Time offers:** These offers induce an urge in the customer to buy a service or product. High-pressure selling pressurizes them by announcing that the service or product might not be available at a later date. Offers made are for a limited duration and urge users through relentless advertisement.

    Have you ever purchased something because it's on sale? Have you made a buying decision because there was a limited time to make a decision? People need a reason to make a buying decision. If not, we procrastinate. It usually happens when people have uncertainty. Uncertainty is fear. Of course, they have fear, who wouldn't be scared to get a procedure? One of the first questions I ask in the consultation is, "How long have you been thinking about it?" "All the time," is the answer or "forever."

Women put themselves last on the list. We are nurturers and caregivers by nature, everyone before ourselves, which is why when they come in considering something for themselves, they've been thinking about it for months and sometimes years. So, if me giving them a timeline and/or a financial incentive is high pressure, well, then I'm all for it. Check, check, and check!

It's all how you see yourself. We were asked to coach a consultant not too long ago in California. She was struggling with getting patients signed up, and the practice manager contacted us for some support. One of the first things she said to me before we started coaching is, "People don't like sales, and neither do I."

"OK, tell me why."

"I never want the patient to feel pushed."

"OK. What do you want them to feel?"

"I want them to want it for themselves, and feel like I'm helping them."

"OK, that's great. Do you believe you're helping them?"

"Yes."

"Do you believe that when a potential patient comes in and shares with you that they want a procedure that you can help them? And you believe in your doctor?"

"Yes, he's great."

"Do you ever have patients that you think are stalling?"

"All the time."

"Why is that?"

"Fear mostly."

"Do you think a good consultant should help them get past their fears?"

"Yes."

"What about the pricing, is that ever an obstacle?"

"Yes."

"Scheduling?"

"Yes."

"Support?"

"Yes."

"Can you help the patient overcome those challenges?"

"Yes."

"So here's what I believe the person that has the problem with sales is you, not the patients. You are in this role to help these people, so help them. Sometimes that means figuring out their budget, sometimes it's holding their hand, and sometimes it's pushing them out of their comfort zone. Does that make sense? We don't call ourselves sales consultants, were coaches. We've changed the title, but be clear, sales is not a bad thing. If you have integrity and empathy and enthusiasm and BELIEF, everything that makes selling so great, you should be proud. Change your paradigm and watch and see if you don't see a difference."

The following month the number of patients scheduled skyrocketed, and that meant her sales did too.

CHAPTER 24: You Can't Make This Stuff Up

Human Resources always have the best stories. When you're dealing with people, you're bound to have problems, and the more people, the more problems. We had some amazing employees, but those are never as fun to reminisce about. I'm talking about the ones when you say, "Remember when..."

As we started to grow rapidly, the issues grew just as fast. I was never a fan of terminations, but it was constant. I always see articles about what companies do wrong—look at websites like Glassdoor. I want to start a company on employee reviews. Why is it you have to be careful with what you say when an employer calls? Only say whether they are eligible for re-hire. How about we tell them all the things the employee did? The employee was stealing from the company. Having inappropriate relations with a coworker. Stole the doctor's prescription pad and wrote scripts. Bartering with a dentist trading a facelift for some new veneers. There were so many you couldn't keep up. We did disc profiles and background checks, but at the rate of growth we had and filling positions at different levels, it was tough to keep up. I used to say, "I should write a book called '*You Just Can't Make This ...Up.*

I remember one manager who was doing some pretty shady stuff. I uncovered and tracked what was happening and followed the appropriate documentation. On the day we went in to terminate her, I had HR fly in to do the termination with me. We knew it wouldn't be pretty. When I told her we were releasing her from her position, she screamed, "You both are total losers, and I should spit on you."

The HR partner calmly said, "And if you do that, we will call the police."

I have escorted many a rage-filled employee out the door. I had one company I worked for a few years back that had a front desk tell the team she was going to hurt herself and was going crazy inside the clinic. We called the police, got her out, and put a restraining order on her. She was continuously calling the employees, and they were scared. I made the decision to close the clinic and have the locks changed. HR called me and asked why I would close the office because we had three cool sculpting treatments that day.

"You're kidding me, right? Yes, I closed the office."

We ended up getting the employee mental health treatment, and she was released soon after. The nurse resigned that night, and I followed quickly behind her. When a company questions why you would close when the team is shaken like that says a lot.

We were constantly interviewing. We had to. We were busy, and I mean busy like no time for a bathroom break. It was full of 'I'm likely to have a UTI from holding it so long' type of days. The candidates would come in droves.

I remember one of the doctors saying, "Wow, I've never seen anything like this. They just keep coming." Our commercials were running nationally, and we were everywhere. We would sometimes have to double and triple up consultations. There was energy in the air, and everyone got it.

Interviewing was fun. It was often done in a hotel lobby. Somedays, we would interview 20-30 candidates. I felt like Simon Cowell on American Idol. We had to make decisions quickly—you've got five minutes. Go.

I remember making a hire down in South Florida. I was sitting in the lobby, she peeked around the corner, touched my shoulder, and said, "I am Maria, when do I start?" Her Spanish accent was thick, and her smile and energy introduced her. She loved everything about plastic surgery and helping women look and feel their best. I hired her on the spot, and she stayed with the company for years as a top consultant.

CHAPTER 25: Who's Got Lunch?

Private practices and doctors' offices are typically closed for lunch for an hour. We were too busy. There weren't enough hours in the day. It was difficult to staff, train, coach, and keep up with everyone. People were working hard, and it was wearing on them. It wasn't until a lawsuit was brought up that addressed overtime violations that we made scheduling changes and started requiring employees to take breaks.

That didn't mean lunch breaks for management, however. There were few exceptions unless you count breakroom meetings that included food. I never once left an office in the forty-eight weeks a year I traveled. It just wasn't done. The company was paying a lot of money for us to fly to a city and pay for a hotel. We needed to be in the office when it opened and when it closed. We were an extension of the team. We were responsible for that office doing well.

I remember a new director was hired and flew out to meet us at the opening of a new location.

"You guys want to go to lunch? There's a great place overlooking the bay. It's only about 35 minutes away."

My colleague and I looked at each other and laughed. Is he kidding? He came from a corporate environment where people in management go out to lunch. We work until the last patient is served or until the sun goes down. I couldn't understand what value it brought for someone to fly to an office, sit in an office on their laptop, take a two-hour lunch, make a couple of observations, and leave.

"I'm sorry. You are making three times the amount than the front desk coordinator, scheduler, and surgical tech make combined, and I'm just wondering what value you bring to the table? At least bring the team some food, but you're more concerned with what you're eating for lunch."

And there you have it... leadership at its finest. I'll stick with the office team and work through lunch.

CHAPTER 26: The Truth Will Set You Free

Why are those people holding signs? I glance out the dusty blinds. Ok, remind me to let the cleaning crew know these are nasty. They are Picketers. Picketing what? Us. Why? Some lady wants her money back? She had her procedure and isn't happy. Okay... have we sat down and talked to her? Has the doctor seen her? Does she need a touch-up or revision? She come in and talked to anyone?

I talked to my fair share of unhappy people. Remember, we did around 200,000 procedures, so you can bet we had some patients that were less than satisfied. I'm not saying we didn't have some less than results; we did. However, I do know that our medical director and team stayed on top of every patient.

Typically, the issue would come from either 1. A doctor that needed training. 2. A patient that didn't comply. I sat through mediations, and I can't tell you how many people don't follow instructions. Smoking was the most common.

I remember early on, a lady sitting across from me, yelling she wanted her money back because she had a poor outcome.

"OMG! What's going on with her face? She has necrosis.[10] She's a smoker. OMG!" I was holding back tears. "She looks awful." I had never seen anything like that before. In fact, it was at that moment I realized I didn't know much except what I was told in training. I knew from training patients were supposed to quit smoking two weeks prior to the procedure, sometimes a month or longer, depending on the surgery.

This woman had an infection after her facelift. She never quit smoking. During

[10] the death of most or all of the cells in an organ or tissue due to disease, injury, or failure of the blood supply.

her procedures, a portion of the blood vessels carry blood to the area, are severed on purpose. Patients who smoke or use nicotine related products have insufficient blood flow, which prevents tissue from getting enough oxygen to survive. This results in the destruction of tissue and/or the inability to heal properly. It can also lead to wound healing problems or even loss of large amounts of skin in a process called necrosis.

I attended several mediations as a representative of Lifestyle Lift; many were from smokers.

So, here's the deal, if you're currently a smoker and thinking about undergoing a cosmetic procedure, you need to stop. This is non-negotiable. Besides that, it's 2019 and should know better. Stop **smoking**! That is all.

"Ma'am, I understand you're upset; it's upsetting for all of us. We had a conversation, and you signed an agreement that you would not smoke."

"I quit smoking. I don't smoke."

"Ma'am, with all due respect, you came in here smelling like an ashtray. I'm asking you to be honest. Can tell me you haven't had any cigarettes before, during, or after your procedure?"

She looked at her husband. "He smokes."

"What about you?" The mediator looked like a deer in headlights and stares back at me. I respond, "No cigarettes?"

"No."

"None? You're a former smoker?"

"Yes."

"How many years did you smoke?"

"Since I was 16."

"Okay, so you've smoked for over 50 years."

"Yes."

"What made you decide to quit?"

"Well-- I-- I just did."

"Ok. Did you quit cold turkey?"

"No, I cut back."

"So, we're going on record here in the courthouse with the mediator that you haven't smoked a cigarette in the last let's say three months. Do you want that on record? Because I'm willing to, in good faith today, provide you with a partial refund that will cover any charges that come with a touch-up. I'm not happy with your results, and I can speak for the doctor when I say I'm sure he isn't either. But we're also talking about a doctor's reputation on the line and whether or not the result was from our negligence or yours. I'm prepared to take this to court if necessary because I believe you have been smoking based on the track record of our surgeon, post-op photos, and what I'm seeing right here today. So, I'll ask one last time."

I looked her in the eye and no response. I looked her husband in the eyes, and he loudly burst out, "She never quit smoking!"

Well, damn, Bob. If looks could kill, she was giving him the look. All women know the look I'm talking about. The mediator shook his head and closed his file. We will offer you a small partial payment, because it's the right thing to do. Thank you both for your time. I shook their hands and walked out of the room.

CHAPTER 27: Just Say No

"Michelle's doing a great job turning our offices around."

"Come on, all she does is go in and sprinkle her little fairy dust. There's no way those offices can sustain those high numbers, we need someone in charge that can keep us consistent at that level."

When I was told these comments made about me from an executive, I worked for I thought, "wow, what nice choice words coming from a man who has tanked several companies, had sexual harassment suits against him and an overall less than stellar professional record." In my mind I was thinking, "Say whatever you want, your opinion of me and my work is hurtful, I'd be lying if I said it wasn't, but I will choose to ignore it and keep pushing on because 1. It's not true 2. I believe in my accomplishments and 3. I have zero respect for you. As my teenage niece would say, Boy Bye."

* * *

I have to give a nod to my husband. He works hard and has done well professionally. One amazing benefit as a married couple with not a lot of bills is that you have financial freedom. We don't live beyond our means, and we don't have much debt, so this allows me to avoid the role of being controlled by money. It affords me not to be a "Yes" person.

My heart goes out to the people every day who are stuck with a less than supervisor or boss. You have mouths to feed, mortgage payments, credit card bills, the list goes on, and you're stuck working with a big fat boob. The supervisor who asks you to stay late, and work while they hit the golf course at noon. The boss that you sit and listen to for hours ramble on about nothing you remotely care about, and pretend you're listening.

Someone close to me recently worked for a boss that had minimal experience in his profession and zero experience managing people. His new boss had worked as a club bouncer until a family friend put him in a vice president position at a well-known, family-owned company. Really? Club bouncer to VP? He was so unbelievably threatened by his management team that he would berate them any chance he got to make himself feel important. He would have them do things like sweeping the floor, take out the garbage, file paperwork for hours, almost like a freshman student going through a college fraternity haze.

Now I'm not above any of those tasks. I tell everyone I'd clean toilets if it helps the business and I will but it is the principle behind it. This guy was flexing his authority and power. My friend said every day while his supervisor, (not exactly how he referenced him) was screaming at them about how awful a job they were doing, he would dream of grabbing him by the throat. The final straw was when this guy told him he was hiring too many black people.

"Excuse me? Wait, he didn't say that?"

"Yes!"

"What did you say?"

"I said the same as you, excuse me?"

"OMG, who says that? Did you contact HR?"

"Michelle, it's a family-owned company. HR isn't gonna do anything, plus it's my word against his."

Now let me side bar a minute about this because if you're a white person reading this book this might make you uncomfortable. I've never had a problem talking about race because at the end of the day it's just my opinion and that's not worth more than anyone else's. Here it is; if you're white, you will never understand what it's like to be black. Just like if you're a man you will never understand what it's like for us as women. I personally grew up in a very integrated world, so for me, I didn't experience seeing much racism until I became older. Maybe I just became more observant? Maybe I was surrounded by more ignorance? I would say both are true.

Some people are more closeted with their feelings. I also believe everyone is racist to some extent. Maybe its unconscious but everyone has some bias towards people. Again, this is just my opinion. Whether you understand it or not, White privilege is real. Now, I haven't taught classes on tolerance so I'm going off common sense here but I'm gonna put this in three buckets; If you fall into the "I have a ton of black friends", bucket than your job is to speak up and educate people when you hear or see something from your fellow whities that is prejudice or discriminating. If you fall into bucket "It was different back then, that's just how I was raised or I have a black friend (meaning you know someone black you occasionally speak to and share pleasantries with)" bucket, I would suggest you try spending some real time with people of different races. Maybe try thinking about what comes out of your mouth before you blurt it out? Or, you can try having someone say or do crude and rude things to you or people that you love so you can comprehend how it feels. If you fall into the "You're hiring too many black people" bucket, well... you're just an ass and there's probably no hope for you. Ok back to the story..

My friend knew after that moment it went beyond an unhealthy work environment; these were not people he wanted to work for. The tough situation is what I'm talking about. Walking away from a paycheck isn't always cut and dry. You don't always know what you're getting into, so you have to put your head down and do what you're told until you either lose it and choke your supervisor or find another job.

Now I'm not at all saying you should cause physical harm, of course not. What I'm saying is, when I see news stories about people going postal, I'm not always surprised. People have enough in the world to deal with. If you roll up into work every day and your boss treats you like garbage, don't be surprised when someone loses his or her cool. Thankfully, I'm in a place where I work for myself and choose exactly who I want to give my time too. Back then, I learned to pick my battles and, as they say in business, "play nice in the sandbox." But I didn't have to say yes all the time like the people around me.

Can you imagine if employees could say what they really thought to their supervisors? That would be the best reality show ever.

“Michelle, what I’d like you to do is pull all the data together, put it in the appropriate documents, and have that ready to present to me by tomorrow.”

“Oh yeah, Jeff. Well, I’d like you to stop staring at my chest, use some dental floss, and stop making me do your job, so you can pass it off as yours. That’s what I’d like you to do Jeff.”

If you call yourself a leader, you need to show authenticity, appreciation, respect, integrity, and trust. You need to engage your employees, listen to them, and show them you care and are committed to constant growth for them and the business. If an employee is working with higher-ups that show favoritism, bully, overwork, blame, punish, gossip, micromanage, you can bet it’s just a matter of time before the business implodes. You may ride the wave awhile, but it always catches up eventually.

In regard to that racist jerk, I was proud of my friend who stepped up and said something. He left the job soon after. He knew that speaking up would likely not change the situation but speaking up was the right thing to do. The best part of this story, that guy got caught doing some illegal stuff on the company and ended up getting fired, but the damage he did to that family's brand on many levels could never be repaired.

CHAPTER 28: #Facts

When it comes to plastic surgery, revisions are an unfortunate reality. According to the American Academy of Facial and Reconstructive Plastic Surgery (AAFPRS), the number of revision surgeries doubled since 2017. Approximately one-third of facial plastic surgeons attributed the rise to non-medical staff doing procedures. Why don't you hear about revisions or unhappy patients more often? Every surgeon has a revision policy. Often, improvements are made, and patients' concerns are properly handled. Most plastic surgeons perform less than thirty facelifts a year. Lifestyle Lift doctors were performing thirty a month. Think about that.

I'm not discrediting anyone who had a bad result. I will tell you that during the years I was with the company, we took every patient complaint seriously. We also had a revision policy that was followed. I can't speak to what happened after I left the organization, but I would hope the same. Now there are websites where you can read reviews... be clear that bad reviews can be removed or buried under positive ones. Every insider knows it too. Techie guys run most of those companies' complaints right to the bottom. There are departments for reputation management, so don't be fooled that all docs don't have a few unhappy patients.

You have no idea who's sitting behind that keyboard. I did a 6-month stint with a medical aesthetics company that offered very popular non-surgical services. They offered a service that was marketed everywhere on television. I mean everywhere. It was promoted as the best procedure out there.

On my first day on the job, I fielded twelve calls about that particular procedure. All twelve people were unhappy with their result and had been blown off by the previous person in charge.

"I want my money back. It didn't work!"

For months, I reviewed before and after photos, charts, and notes of hundreds of unhappy people. That doesn't mean it didn't work for some. For many people, the service wasn't positioned correctly where they were sold one treatment when it should have been two or three.

It is important to speak to people that have had the procedure, research the pros and cons, get the facts. That's exactly why I started MyCoachMD. If you're not an insider, you don't know. Think about the career you're in right now. You probably know a lot more than most about whatever it is you do. Little tips and tricks and good to knows. That's exactly why we're in business—to give you the knowledge. Know Before You Go.

CHAPTER 29: Don't Believe the Hype

Right before I left Lifestyle Lift, they were signing Debby Boone to be featured on their infomercial singing her hit song from the late 1970s, *You Light Up My Life*. I was surprised they went in the direction of someone who hadn't had the procedure. I was asked about it regularly. People would say to me, "Yes, that Debbie Boone had an LSL." No, nope, she, in fact, did not. I stopped in to visit one of my former colleagues who was in town for training, and as I took a seat in the lobby, I noticed there was a giant-sized, cheesy cardboard cutout of Debbie in the lobby.

"Do you have these in all the offices?"

He laughed. "Well, yes, we do."

Oh dear. Lifestyle Lift was everywhere.

In the early years, we were disrupting the industry, and we had enemies. It was commonly written and falsely stated that the majority of Lifestyle Lift doctors were not plastic surgeons and were not credible. This couldn't be further from the truth. All of the doctors inside the company were either board-certified or board eligible. Board eligible means they need to complete a certain number of procedures (not just a facelift) before they can sit for their boards.

Why were people writing this stuff? Every patient was given a copy of their doctor's bio, they met their doctors before their surgery—not the day of surgery like many people claimed—and we spoke specifically in the consultation about their doctor's background. That's part of why consultants see the patient first. It gives them a chance to talk about the surgeon in more detail.

Recruiting doctors became easier. I remember one senior gentleman team member who felt the need to compare us to Home Depot ™ and the mom and pop hardware store. He would say they can run their little private practice, or they can join us. We're going to open in their city and take all their patients. I felt like I was in an episode of *The Office.* I was Jim

Halpern when Michael Scott would be speaking. A dead stare is all I could give back. Why would you compare a well-accomplished plastic surgeon who built up his practice to a hardware store? *I hate you.* Yes, that's what I was saying inside my head. Repeatedly. I didn't really hate him. I actually thought he was a decent guy, just an idiot in this business. I believe that was the problem with a lot of the men; they were smart and capable, just not in the aesthetics industry.

It was stated somewhere, and I say somewhere because I can't remember where, that over a period; there were 90 registered complaints against Lifestyle Lift. We performed more than 200,000 procedures. The problem is that the industry and Internet hammered us. I hated that we had even one complaint, but it is a reality and a risk you take when you have any type of procedure.

We had complaints that they hadn't met the doctor before surgery, complaints that we took their money that we would guarantee they would look ten years younger. The facts were that we told them they would look years younger. We told them the procedure lasts years, and "... you will always look younger than if you didn't have it done."

Patients always met the doctor before surgery in a separate appointment. Our business model was set up differently because we offered a free consult. The consultant saw the patient because the doctors were busy in surgery. If they had time that day, they would absolutely come in and meet the patient. We eventually adjusted the model so that most patients would, in fact, see the doctor the same day as their free consult. It was tricky to always do, but we wanted to avoid any concern or confusion on the part of the potential patient. Contrary to what people believed, we really were always working toward improving the patient experience.

In terms of payment, if a potential patient made the decision to schedule, they would be required to put down a small reservation fee. This is no different than a private practice that charges for meeting the plastic surgeon and, just like us, that money was applied to the balance. If the patient canceled outside a specific window on the contract or close to the surgery date, we may not refund. Again, same as any other practice.

During the height of business success, during the years I worked there, we were receiving around 14,000 calls a week. Out of those calls, for the people that booked an appointment, showed up for an appointment, scheduled an appointment, met the doctor, booked a procedure, had a clearance, and made it to surgery, was between 3-4%. People on the outside, especially in the medical field, really had no idea how much work went into driving patient throughput. We had this image that people called, we invited them in and pushed everybody in the chair for a procedure. Not even close.

CHAPTER 30: Price Chopper

You get what you pay for. I could end the chapter here. Very simply put, don't buy on price. I know it's tempting, and I know you want a good deal unless you are drowning in cash and have your plastic surgeon on speed dial. My advice: if you are concerned with price, get two or three quotes. If you go much past that, you're probably never going to get a procedure because you're neurotic and likely going to be a super high-maintenance patient that everyone runs from. FYI, doctors do turn patients away.

I've worked for several national chains that offered affordable procedures. Lifestyle Lift facelifts were about a third lower in price than traditional facelifts.

Pricing was affordable, and that meant more procedures needed to be performed. Meetings were taking place weekly on how many surgeries could be completed by each doctor in a day. We were getting granular with times, supplies, and if we could move up production and capacity, to increase revenue. We had some doctors doing seven procedures a day. It was insane. The younger, faster doctors were celebrated, and the slow docs were talked about behind closed doors. Do we need to replace him? We had some offices that had 3-4 docs, and our staff had preferences. We did have some phenomenal docs, and we had a few that needed training or needed to hit the links because it was time to retire and play golf.

I would get a call from corporate when there was an uneven distribution of cases amongst doctors. The field team saw the variances because of patient complaints, and they spoke up, which was great. There were times doctors needed training, and we could then immediately communicate with our medical director to address. I always told the staff to do the right thing. If that meant uneven distribution of cases, I would take the heat. I didn't always tell corporate that because I knew they wouldn't like that coaching, but in the famous words of a senior team member who gambled regularly on his questionable decisions, "It was a risk I was willing to take."

CHAPTER 31: Somebody's Watching Me

According to data prepared by an LSL financial advisor, at its peak in 2013, the company brought in 186 million in revenues and performed 18% of all facelifts done by board-certified physicians in the United States. The company was continuing to open up locations, and I left and moved on to a Vice President Position of a startup aesthetic company that purchased full-body plastic surgery clinics. The American Association accredited the clinics for Accreditation of Ambulatory Surgery Facilities (AAAASF), which is considered the Gold-Standard in accreditation.

We had outstanding plastic surgeons, and we were working on developing a new brand and business model for everything surgical and non-surgical. I made a point of keeping quiet as to where I was working. I was still connected to quite a few people at Lifestyle Lift when I was advised that someone from the senior management team had hired a private investigator to see if I was stealing trade secrets. I don't know if that was true and thought it was a little extreme if it was. Most of what we trained on or implemented was nothing proprietary. It was my work anyway, but they could have it because you can have all the tools you want; if you don't have the right people to execute, it means nothing.

CHAPTER 32: Stop What You're Doin'

Florida Attorney General Pam Bondi and Lifestyle Lift agreed to change its marketing materials and practices to eliminate any possible consumer confusion about its services in a USA Today article dated 2013.

According to a press release by the Florida Attorney General, As part of the agreement, Lifestyle Lift (LSL) must disclose any compensation made to the models used in its advertisements and its materials, disclose what facial rejuvenation services were performed on models in the company's marketing materials, and comply with Federal Trade Commission guidelines concerning the use of before-and-after photographs of models in endorsements and testimonials in marketing materials. The company has also agreed not to use the term "revolutionary procedure" to describe the basic Lifestyle Lift.

What's more, Florida consumers who purchased services between June 1, 2009, and June 10, 2013, may be entitled to a refund. The Company must also pay Florida's legal fees and contribute $25,000 to a fund called Seniors v. crime. In a press release, the LSL Corporation points out that the Assurance of Voluntary Compliance agreement finds no violation of any state or federal law and is the final resolution of the matter.

In the Assurance of Voluntary Compliance, Attorney General Bondi said that Lifestyle Lift® acted in good faith and found that there was no violation of any state or federal law. There was no penalty or fine. The Attorney General also acknowledged that Lifestyle Lift® had an established process for handling customer satisfaction issues and inquiries.

The takeaway from this was basically to stop saying the procedure was revolutionary, disclose that the patients who become models are paid to use their before and after photographs and increase the font size of all disclaimers. All fair adjustments.

CHAPTER 33: The Greatest Job

I wouldn't write a book without a chapter on being a mom. Maybe it sounds strange to some women, but I never had the desire to be a mom. I had nieces and nephews who I adored, and they gave me that unconditional love that you can only get from being a part of the lives of children. Having my daughter was a surprise, and I always say if I had known how much love I would have felt, I would have had more children, but I was older, and that ship had sailed. I also don't believe if I hadn't made the decision to leave Lifestyle Lift, I would have ever had my daughter. So, I'm thankful that everything happened the way it did.

Being an older mom has its advantages and disadvantages. It's not an easy transition when you go from career to family. I don't know if it's talked about much. You hear about women having postpartum or stay at home moms. What about the workingwomen trying to find themselves and their identity?

When I had my daughter, I was all in. It was love at first sight. What do I do now? Work on the budget, and make a bottle, jump off a conference call and change a diaper. Is this how it's supposed to be? I took about three months off, and I remember going on a play date with some other moms, and the entire conversation was about crying, napping, and safe toys. I couldn't help drifting. I missed the stimulation and the adrenaline rush of working. I had always had a job.

I grew up on a golf course and started selling lemonade during tournaments every summer from the age of 10. That's when I got my first taste of sales. Greet the customer; provide good service and a good product. I'm not sure how good the product was, but how can you not buy lemonade from little girls on the ninth hole sitting in the sun all day watching old men in checkered pants throw clubs? We sold the lemonade for 50 cents, but it wasn't uncommon for them to pay with $1's and $5's. The friendlier we were, the bigger the tip. We would clear $300 a weekend, split between my best friend and me. We were able to buy some cool stonewashed jeans and some jelly bracelets.

When I turned 16, I became a lifeguard and taught swim lessons. I worked throughout the school year at a local high school and the local country club. I would always see the moms lounging by the pool in their wide-brimmed hats and big sunglasses, reading a romance novel while we kept an eye on their little ones. I liked sitting high up in my lifeguard chair in my red bathing suit and whistle. I felt in charge, and I liked observing the members. I would see the same mom's day in and day out and wondered if this was what life was like when you got old. Mind you, I'm probably not much older now than those women were, but when you're a teenager, everyone is old.

Both my parents worked. My mother was one of eight children and the only one to graduate from high school, let alone receive both an undergraduate and a graduate degree. She waited tables while she went to school and spent twenty-five years teaching special education.

My father was a physical education teacher. He coached high school baseball for years before moving over to coach girls' high school softball. My dad, along with all the other coaches in our town, spent the summers working at the prison, running softball tournaments for inmates. He said it wasn't a place he wanted to be, but they paid well.

I never saw my parents not putting in the hustle, so I'm sure seeing them as examples impacted me as well. Because my mom went to school during the day and waited tables at night, my sister and I were raised in a gym, school bus, and dugout. I learned to score a baseball game by the time I was nine. We had most dinners at McDonalds and Burger King coming back from a game with the team. I can't remember a time I wasn't around sports. If I wasn't watching sports or working as a lifeguard and swim coach, I was playing summer travel ball.

When I came home from college, I spent my Christmas breaks working mall retail and summers working for the US Postal Service as a summer mail carrier. We would start our mornings at 5:30 am casing the mail, bundling it, then out on the truck to start our routes. Summer carriers always got the hardest routes. The old-timers would take the riding routes and leave the 10-14mile a day treks to the summer help. I had a job throughout college where all my friends and I worked in one giant room with cubicles. Our job was to call people from a phonebook and ask them political questions. For every survey completed we got $3 plus our hourly wage of $8. We didn't take it seriously, but we had a lot of fun.

Right out of college, I took a job in my field of social work, working with the mentally disabled. While that job takes a special person, it was definitely not for me. There wasn't much opportunity in a small town, and I ended up taking a temporary job in a factory. It was eight hours of repetition, day in and day out. It was all about speed and accuracy.

We would get new products to package every week, and these people grinded. We would punch a time clock 30-minute lunch break, two 15-minute breaks, and then back on the line. We wore hairnets and would sweat through our shirts. Most of the people would chain smoke cigarettes on their break. I would think to myself, while following the conveyor belt, how do people do this? Are they happy? They seemed nice and content. There wasn't much time for talking, which was very difficult for me. If you messed up the line, production goes down, and that meant money lost.

A few weeks in, I was moved to the big time-packing film. This paid another $1 an hour and was no joke. It was a big contract with Kodak, and you didn't want to screw up and have those machines go down. If you made that line you, had factory cred. These people walked around like they owned the place. This was an entirely new level of work. We had more freedom to talk because of the pace, and the people were hysterical. They didn't hold anything back, and the stories they told are an entirely separate book. I learned to hold six rolls of film at once; three in each hand, as we carefully dropped into packaging every few seconds. It had a fast pace, and it felt like the game beat the clock for hours. I don't know how someone could do it for longer than a few months, but it was better than what I had been doing.

Some of the people had been there for 40 years. After my month on the film line, I was approached by the supervisor and offered a full-time position with higher hourly and benefits. I remember thinking, is this what I'm going to do? I remember walking to the time clock when one of the ladies walked next to me.

She said, "Honey, you got a college degree, right?"

"Yes."

"You don't need to be working on the line. If you take it, you might get stuck. You got more to offer."

I smiled and said, "Thank you."

I walked into the supervisor's office the next morning and declined the job. I asked if there were any other positions available. The next day I started as the switchboard operator.

At the front of the house, I saw all the comings and goings. The owner's daughter held a high position, and there were two other women in management—the rest were men. I was answering phones and listening in on business conversations when I could. I was bored. When a position came up in customer service, I went immediately to my supervisor's office. I'd like to apply for the customer service position.

"Michelle, you're doing great on the phones, the best we've had. That customer service position is too much for you."

Pause...what did he just say to me? "I don't understand Bob, I have a four-year degree, and I've held customer service positions before working retail."

"Yeah, you're just fine sitting pretty right where you are. Oh, the phone's ringing you need to get back to your seat."

I resigned two weeks later.

I took a pit stop career move at a fitness club. I made protein shakes and sold gym memberships. I landed my first "real job" at State Farm Insurance as a claims adjuster.

It's funny the things you remember. One of the guys at the gym told me that they were hiring, and the only requirement was a 4-year degree. I immediately sent in my resume and had an interview by end of week. I remember being ridiculously nervous. I walked in and took a seat with a long line of other applicants. The interview was done by a panel, and we were told they were hiring four new reps. I kept thinking, keep your eye on the ball, focus.

The door opened and out walked one of the guys from the gym. This guy was so cocky. I said, "Hello."

"Oh, Hey Michelle, what are you doing here?"

I'm just hanging out in the state farm lobby. "Same reason that you're here, Kevin."

"Cool."

"How'd it go in there?"

"Oh, it's in the bag."

"I should just leave then, huh?"

He laughed and tapped my leg. "Hey, good luck. See ya at the gym tomorrow. You can have my shake ready."

I said some choice words under my breath and put my head down. When they called my name, my nerves were gone. Kevin had actually done me a favor. At that point, I was of the mindset he got the job, so I've got nothing to lose anyway.

I got a call a few days later that I got the job. Of course, I couldn't let it go, so I made sure to tell Kevin when I saw him at the gym that my position at the gym was now open, and I would put in a good word for him.

State Farm was a great job. The other three reps that were hired at the same time as me are still working there 20+ years later. One is still one of my best friends.

As solid as State Farm was, a friend landed a job where she was making some serious money. She told me she was working for a software company start-up and, they were hiring. I went in for an interview and landed the job. When I told my boss, he was upset.

It was hard to get into State Farm, and they invest a lot of money into training and retaining their employees. We spent months learning policy. We had completed fire claims school at their corporate headquarters in Illinois, where they had model homes set up with all different types of scenarios, so you could practice how to inspect and investigate. My favorite was theft claims. We would get to take hundreds of recorded statements and had to escalate quite a few to our special investigative unit. It's quite amazing how many women lose their diamond rings scuba diving on their honeymoons.

State Farm wasn't a job you leave. I remember my boss writing down a dollar amount on a piece of paper, and saying, "I will guarantee you this in two years, plus a management position if you stay."

I looked at the number and looked back at him. "I really appreciate the offer. I'm gonna have to take a shot at this new opportunity."

I spent the next two years selling customized help desk and project management software to businesses over the phone. Our developer would fly out to do onsite presentations, and we would travel for trade shows. We all got company cars and made big commission checks. I really didn't know what I was doing, but I knew how to talk to people, so I would do the talking and let my colleague do the demos.

I stayed there until I moved to NYC, where I worked basically right out of the movie boiler room doing sales with about 300 25-year-old men in cheap suits. There were four girls on the floor, and we sold luxury retreats to CEOs. If you were lucky enough to get past the secretary gatekeeper and get a sale, you got to ring the bell in the middle of the floor. It was fun.

After some time in NY, I spent time in Washington, D.C., where I worked for the U.S. Chamber of Commerce selling chamber memberships. From there, I moved back home and decided to open an ice cream shop. Again, that's another story for another book.

Next, a quick pit stop working at a bank. They hired me as a relationship manager, which was basically bringing in lunch and dropping off pens to their accounts. After three months, I made an appointment with the President of the bank.

"I appreciate the opportunity; however, I'm not challenged and could do more."

The next week he moved me to a Mortgage originator position until I eventually moved to my longer-term stop entering the weight loss industry.

I've had a job my entire life. It's what I know. Now I have a baby who needs me, and I need to take care of. Who's going to hire me, and do I even want to work? I had just finished working with a small aesthetics company start-up, and I wasn't sure what was next, so I just decided to give myself time to regroup. Within a week, I got a call from a company that found me on LinkedIn and wanted me to fly overseas to meet with some investors on a new plastic surgery venture. One thing about a good reputation and industry experience, I no longer had to interview.

Not too long ago, someone asked if I had a resume. I had to stop and think about it. No? Not since 2005. I decided that I was potentially interested, but wasn't comfortable with flying, so they came to me. The next few years were some of the best in my career. I wouldn't say it was easy, but with the help of my family, I was able to make it work.

In my next position, I worked a schedule that allowed me to take my daughter to school and pick her up most days. I can say I've never missed a recital, swim meet, school play, or anything that I know she would want mom for.

Being at a level in my career where I could forge my own path felt like validation for all the years of hard work. I spent years as an independent consultant with different companies that allowed me the ability to be a mom and a working professional.

I knew that I had to stay relevant, stay in the industry if I was ever going to build my own company, but I had to do it on my terms. I had so many people say, "You're so lucky they let you work that schedule." That wasn't luck that was industry credibility, high performance results and years at the grind. Now I've got a new grind. Working mom.

I can't understand why more companies don't get it. Moms are it; they are the boss. Are you kidding me? Find a good mom trait and tell me if it doesn't fall under leadership.

1. Patience... that should be listed twice
2. Empathy
3. Multitasker
4. Problem Solver
5. Resilience
6. Self-Control

7. Sense of Humor
8. Fearlessness
9. Humility
10. Celebration
11. Care
12. Persuasion
13. Compassion

Let me tell you something; companies are missing the boat not hiring more working mothers. As a mom, I was even better, more in control. I easily saw the benefits of work smarter, not harder. Please, I can make a bottle, change a dirty diaper, take a call all at the same time? I can do anything.

My professional dream is to keep building a ridiculous pool of female talent together that allows them the ability to make a living and a life. It's why you see so many of these multi-level marketing companies. Women want to support themselves and each other, they want to bring money to the table, and they want to be part of something bigger that they can utilize their experience and skills. They also want to excel highly at their number one job, and that's being a mom.

CHAPTER 34: Phone a Friend

"Who's supporting you in the decision, Mary?"

"Nobody."

"Does your husband know you're here?"

"No, and I'm not going to tell him."

"Well, I want you to know there is a recovery period. If you are living under the same roof, he's definitely going to know, and you need someone after the procedure."

"He travels out of the country for work, so I want to do it then."

"Ok, who then will help support you?"

"I don't know. I don't really have anyone."

"Well, who's your go-to? Who's the first person you call when you leave here today, you're first on speed dial?"

"That's Karen, my best friend, and next-door neighbor. She lives in the condo right next to me, and we play *Bridge* every Thursday. There's a group of us, and we have a great time. We make martinis and play out on my sunporch. I swear she's had this done, but she says no!"

"Well, she wouldn't be the first woman to deny having work done! Are you comfortable telling her?"

"Yes, I don't care if she knows, I just don't want Jim to know because he won't want me to spend the money even though he buys whatever he wants and has three different golf memberships! You know what I do; I leave my bags in the car when I go shopping if his car is in the garage. I don't want him asking me questions about how much I spent. I'm retired. I've worked and raised three children, are you kidding me?"

"Do you have separate accounts?"

"No, but I pay all the credit card bills. If I really wanted it, he wouldn't care. I just don't want to get the third degree, so I'll just tell him after."

"What about your children? Will you tell them?"

"Just my daughters. My son will tell me no. I don't know why; his wife has had a tummy tuck and her boobs done!"

"So, when Jim is traveling, we need Karen to step in and support you. You need someone with you overnight."

"Oh, that's not a problem. Let me call her right now; she's probably out shopping or at her aerobics class."

Here's their conversation:

"Hi Karen, it's Mary. Can you spend the night with me on the 25th? I'm getting a facelift? I need you to drive me to and from and stay with me a couple of nights while Jim is out of town. Yes, Karen, a facelift. Karen, please, everyone knows you had one too! Yes, you did. Will you do it or not? I'm here with this nice young lady, and we're looking at the schedule."

She covers the speaker of her phone with her right hand, "You're so darling by the way, how old are you?"

I smile. "Thank you. 33," I whisper.

"Just a baby!" Back to Karen. "Yes, your dog Mitzi can come too." Mary rolls her eyes. "Yes, he's board-certified. No, I don't know if he's single. Jesus, Karen, will you do it or not? I'm handing the phone to Michelle."

"Hi Karen, this is Michelle. I work with the doctor. Yes, she's in great hands. Dr. Z is board practicing for over 18 years, and he's board-certified in facial plastic surgery. He actually just met with her, and she's coming back next week for her formal pre-operative visit. We'd love for you to come! It's next Tuesday. Yes, I will be here. No, he is not single, but we do have a lot of single men who come in for procedures, so I can definitely keep on the lookout for you! Yes, Mary said you are very attractive and in great shape for your age. You do aerobics, right?" I laugh and put the speaker to my chin.

"Karen, she said quit sharing her personal business! I'd love to meet you with Karen, are you free next Tuesday at 10? Great! Mary, does that work for you?"

"Yes, and tell her I will take her to lunch after."

"Mary is taking you out to lunch after for taking care of her. Looking forward to meeting you. Thank you. Here's Mary."

Mary and Karen came in together that Tuesday. They were in the office for three hours, making everyone laugh. Mary had her procedure. She was bruised for two weeks, but by week three, she was looking good. I would have normally seen her at her 30-day follow up visit, however she stopped in to see us since she was Karen's driver. Karen decided to schedule an upper and lower eye procedure the day she came in to support Mary. Karen said there was no way she could have Mary looking better than her. Those two beauties were unforgettable.

It's imperative when you have a surgical procedure to have someone to support you. If you have a procedure that doesn't require a hospital stay, you do need someone to be with you overnight. You would be surprised how many people say they have someone and don't. Waivers are required to be signed, and at one company, we ended up having to implement a new policy to have a signature for the driver, and the patient would not be released until we had the driver sign off acknowledging they were the patient's driver while the patient was in the car.

We had a family member drop off his father for a body contouring procedure under local anesthesia. They signed the transportation forms and left. We had no idea the family member was leaving the car and being picked up, having no plans to stay with their father. When the procedure is completed, there is a period where the patient would rest in a wheelchair. The nurse removed the IV and gave him some apple juice. The nurse asked about his ride, and he said they were waiting outback. He then asked for another apple juice. She went into the adjacent room, turned around, and he was gone.

It was not uncommon for patients who had procedures under local to be up and around while others had stronger effects to medication. This guy made a run for it. The nurse thought maybe he went to the restroom. She went to the nurse's station, where I was chatting with one of the girls.

"Did you guys just see my patient walk by?"

"No, Mark?"

"Yes."

"No, he hasn't been here. He's done with surgery, right?"

"Yes, and he was sitting in his wheelchair and then disappeared. I literally turned my back for a minute to get him something to drink."

"Everything go well?"

"Yes, great. He said he felt fine."

"Oh no."

We walked to the front. Mark was nowhere to be found. We had barely gotten two steps when our front desk coordinator said, "Michelle, Mark is on the phone." I made a face like 'No, he didn't!'

"Mark, where are you?!"

"Michelle, I'm so sorry! I know it's against policy, and I don't want to get anyone in trouble. I feel fine."

"You're not fine, Mark. You've taken medication, and it's a liability to have you behind the wheel."

"I'm a big guy. I'm fine. I feel fine, really. My daughter couldn't wait, and I knew if I told you, I couldn't have my procedure today."

"There are so many things wrong with this and my god if anything happens—"

"I'm fine. I'm driving slowly, almost there. Please don't be mad. Everyone there is so nice."

At this point, most of the team is gathered around me.

"How far are you?"

"10 minutes. I'm staying on the phone with you."

"Where are you going?"

"A friend's house."

"So much for a friend that couldn't pick you up?"

I stayed on the phone, and Mark got to his friend's house safely. I spoke with his friend, who assured me he would stay with him overnight. The doctor called him later and was nicer than I was. Thankfully, Mark was safe.

I've met with a lot of people over the years who don't have help but want procedures. There are so many great services out there that provide assistance and overnight care. Whichever doctor you choose, they will likely have a list of providers that can help support you. In addition to the physical support, you likely need some emotional support. Plastic surgery can be a roller coaster of emotions. It's not like a before and after show when you see them going in and then fast-forward through a few commercials to the big reveal. There's a lot of time in between, and it's another reason why my partners and I started MyCoachMD. We want to make sure you are not only educated on procedure options and get you in front of qualified, board-certified docs, but we also want to provide you the emotional support and encouragement.

Your mindset plays a big part in your experience and outcome. We did a study while I was at one company that determined most patient complaints were about how they were made to feel. Not the result, how they felt. “I felt like they didn’t care, I felt rushed, I felt dismissed with my concerns.” This is the part that is so bothersome. What may be a small concern with a strange lump they felt or concern about swelling can escalate to an awful experience, which, in turn, can move to an online review and a bad reputation. If you’re a doctor, own a practice or any business for that matter, how you make someone feel is just as important as the outcome really. Take care of people, address their concerns, and validate their feelings and you will reduce the complaints received from customers in any field of expertise.

CHAPTER 35: Sweet Emotion

Did you know that there are 27 different categories of emotions? Different types of emotions that influence how we interact and live our lives, how we respond, engage and make decisions.

Everyone displays his or her emotions differently. For me I've always been drawn to someone who shows outward expression. One of my favorites is intensity, especially of an athlete. I don't care if its golf, tennis, football-the display of energy and concentration...to me there is nothing better than a winning, arm raised high in the air, fist pump. I'm not talking about the jersey shore fist pump (although those are pretty awesome too,) I'm talking about Serena Williams's center court. An awe-inspiring athlete with both physical and mental strength. (If by any chance Serena you are reading this book, you are my girl crush) the power and strength, and precision that go into her work after an intense volley... and when that moment of the victory hits intensity-YES!! Nothing better. Whether it's a jump up and down, a victory dance or fist pump, I love that shot of adrenaline, that makes you feel good kind of emotion.

On the opposite spectrum comes around the emotion of sadness. For the older demographic patients, I've met with you could probably throw in a bit of shame, embarrassment, and fear. These are the types of emotions that often come into my world when I'm coaching. My goal is to move that sadness to the opposite of the spectrum.

She looks in the mirror. Watching her slowly turn her neck from side to side. Raising her hands to her face, she presses and slides her fingertips along her jawline and pulls her skin towards her ears. She moves next to her neck, almost as if she's grabbing her throat. She lifts up on her eyelids. "I look so tired and old. Who is this person, I don't recognize myself? It's not that I want to look different, I just want to look a little better, I want to look like me, just less tired and refreshed."

I've looked into those same eyes more than I can count.

How would you feel as a young woman to look in the eyes of women twice your age every day? Who tell you that they've stayed in marriages faithfully for years until one day out of the blue their husband left them for a younger woman? Who told you that they've outlived their children? They've worked forty years at the same job, waiting tables or in the factory. They've lived through house fires, car accidents, weddings and funerals. These same women have travelled the world and those who have never left their hometowns. Women who have folded countless piles of laundry and had dinner on the table every night at six o'clock since they were twenty-one... sitting across from a women who tells you, looking you in the eyes, sitting in front of you, that when she looks at herself in the mirror she doesn't like what she sees. These beautiful women with incredible stories and with years of aging to show for it. Now for some women, this doesn't bother them, but for many, the ones that come to us, it does.

The woman that wants to find herself again, to bring back her vigor and that sparkle in her eye. She wants hope, a boost, and a transformation to feel alive again. Would you want to help them? Because when I look into her eyes, I want to help.

I want to help because I see myself. I see you. Because whether your 29, 49 or 70, whether you walk the red carpet or work on the assembly line, you DESERVE to look and feel good. If that means the stories of these women who are looking for facial rejuvenation or patients looking for something else, whatever it is that could play even a small part in moving that emotion away from sadness. Everyone deserves to be happy.

For every single woman that has trusted me with their personal story, thank you. Thank you for educating me on life. What I learned as a young woman from the thousands of mothers and grandmothers that passed along so much wisdom, I was given this key takeaway and I'll pass the wisdom on to all of you. Love yourself first.

You can be a great wife, mother, daughter, sister, colleague, or friend. But do not, and I mean do not forget about yourself along the way. Don't put your needs aside because the roof needs to be fixed or that theirs another weekend soccer tournament... life moves fast my friend, and you deserve to make yourself a priority too.

CHAPTER 36: #Facts Part 2

I was saddened to find this online: Plastic-surgery chain Lifestyle Lift filed for Chapter 11 protection Friday, 3½ weeks after abruptly shutting down its business and laying off its staff of nearly 400.

The filing, in U.S. Bankruptcy Court in Detroit, lists assets of less than $50,000 and liabilities of between $10 million and $50 million.

Lifestyle Lift said it is negotiating with a new management company to reopen most, if not all, of its roughly 50 centers. The new company "is hoping to rehire the former employees at those centers, including doctors and medical staff."

"All possible actions are being taken to ensure the preservation and privacy of the patient medical records," Lifestyle Lift said.

The company, which filed for bankruptcy along with several related entities, owes money to vendors including Botox maker Allergan Inc.

Its debts include $17.4 million due to J.P. Morgan Chase & Co. and $5.5 million owed to a former investor, Mark Mitchell, who successfully sued the company to recoup his investment, according to filings.

In addition, more than a dozen people have sued the company, some who appear to be former employees and patients, court filings show. Most of the litigation is listed as pending, with the amount of liability to be determined.

Founded in 2001 by Dr. David Kent, Lifestyle Lift pioneered the mass marketing of plastic surgery through its nationwide chain of surgery centers. It's marketing touted face-lift procedures that, unlike most cosmetic surgery, required only local anesthesia.[11]

---

[11] The Wall Street Journal; March 27, 2015; Sara Randazzo; https://www.wsj.com/articles/plastic-surgery-chain-lifestyle-lift-seeks-bankruptcy-protection-1427504308

CHAPTER 37: The Comeback

I didn't know 15 years ago I would be working in plastic surgery. I certainly didn't think I would be writing a book about it. They say if you can get paid doing something you're passionate about, then you got it right. Having been in the field of aesthetics for years, we know that every client is unique and wants to be confident in their decisions.

Our mission at MYCoachMD is to offer inspiration and empowerment. We don't replace the doctor consultation, and we don't give medical advice; we simply educate and help people evaluate their options on cosmetic services, procedures, pricing financing, and a list of doctors that meet specific criteria. Once they make a decision for themselves, we work with the practices to provide ongoing coaching and support so that every patient can have a great experience.

As the CEO of MYCoachMD, We are building a team of awesome people who want to coach and connect. We promised ourselves we wouldn't make decisions based on money whether we stay small or grow ridiculously big. We want to make sure we are always bringing value and making a positive connection and impact

We had a few twists and turns along the way. We started with some great partners who had a different vision, and after some time, we mutually decided to part ways. In the past, I may have made my decision on loyalty to others. Today, I make decisions that are loyal to me. I no longer ignore my gut feelings, and I also don't stay longer than I should if I know something isn't right.

In addition to MyCoachMD, my partners and I operate The Plastic Surgery Coach. We offer coaching to other Patient Coordinators and Doctors. We've been very fortunate to have an ongoing steady stream of clients. We've talked about a long-term goal of scaling, but if we don't, that's ok too. We've learned so much along the way, and though it's still exciting to climb the mountain if getting to the top means compromising our happiness, we're not interested. We agreed early on that we would be open to new opportunities and follow the unchartered path as long as it is done our way.

A few months back, I received a call from Dr. Kent. We had stayed in touch through the years, and I went to him from time to time for advice on my business. I was building my business, and he was rebuilding his. I knew he had gone through some pretty tough personal struggles in additional to his professional loss.

I had heard toward the end of Lifestyle Lift he was a different person. I would imagine that anyone who has that level of success and a complete 360-life transition would be affected in ways we couldn't likely understand. He was my friend, and anyone who knows me knows, if you are my friend, you're family.

On our periodic calls, Dr. Kent always asked how my father is doing. Over the years, he had sent my father a couple of books on coaching. My father was my chauffeur for my entire six years at Lifestyle Lift. He is a retired teacher and coach and wanted to make a little side money, so I had him pick me up and drop me off at the airport all those weeks I traveled the country for Lifestyle Lift. I laugh because we really should have put him on the payroll. There was nothing he didn't know about the company and the inner workings.

At my wedding, Dr. Kent flew in on his private plane with a few other close friends who were coworkers. My dad had given a toast and during the speech, referenced my years at Lifestyle Lift. He talked about my work ethic, love, and dedication for that company. After the speech, my dad saw Dr. Kent in the hallway and pulled him aside. Of course, I am my father's child.

"Let me tell you something, David, if you don't already know, Michelle is the hardest working and loyal person you will ever have in your company. She could run your company."

Dr. Kent smiled. "I know she can!"

It's funny how life takes you in different directions. My parents are the biggest influencers in my life. My dad will tell you that God has given him the gift of discernment, and he has passed that trait on to me. Recently, when Dr. Kent called me and asked me to take on his start-up business as a client I it knew it was the right decision. I talked it over with my business partners and said yes. As long as we can still keep MyCoachMD as our primary focus.

Everyone loves a comeback story. It takes some serious courage and resilience to get back up again. But they say the win is sweeter after the fall. From a business standpoint, I don't care who you are, I have respect for anyone going for it. It takes a lot of resilience and mental strength. Two traits I highly respect.

And just like we root for the comeback, the comeback doesn't happen alone. It takes the heart of the people, a community that draws strength from each other. I believe this is what no money or power or greed can touch. The comeback starts by showing up, and here

I am, as the coach. Whatever happens, I'm having fun, and I'm going for the win.

Chapter 38: Everyone Needs a Coach

The aesthetic industry continues to evolve, however one thing that stays constant is a person need for growth. More and more people are relying on a coach for guidance. People know what they want, sometimes need support, accountability or an extra nudge to make it happen. As coaches, if we can help others with positive change that will result in greater fulfillment, personally or professionally, well that's pretty awesome.

My colleagues and I are all about establishing a trust-based relationship to help achieve goals, answer questions, identify roadblocks, and ultimately bring out the best in people, inspiring them to take action towards transformation. We are committed to the empowerment of others by bridging the gap between where you are today and where you want to be tomorrow. We work with people one on one to provide a personalized experience. If that means working with a doctor that struggles with connecting with patients, or a woman that has always thought about plastic surgery but is scared, or the patient that's had a procedure and is feeling alone going through the emotional journey, were here to hold your hand, answer questions, support and lift you up, whatever we can do to help create a great patient experience, that is our goal.

The work we do goes beyond following a set of policies and procedures, fitting into the corporate "boys club", or collecting a paycheck. It's not about how much money is made or how many degrees you have hanging on the wall. It's not about if you live in the Hollywood Hills or in a small town in Idaho. It's not white-collar or blue-collar; it's about all people living an

Engaged

Meaningful

And Happy life, to me that is everything. That is all.

If you have questions or are considering plastic surgery or you are a doctor or practice that needs support and guidance on to create a great patient experience for your patients, we can help.

Everyone needs a coach.

Let's get started.

www.mycoachmd.com

About the Author

With close to two decades of experience in the field of aesthetics, Michelle Emmick, also Known as The Plastic Surgery Coach has taken her stories to paper writing her first novel Blue-Collar Beauty, Confessions of a Plastic Surgery Coach. Michelle has performed over 10,000 patient consultations and trained over 3000 doctors and support staff in the US and Internationally. Michelle's writing style is no-nonsense, comical and heartfelt with insider stories that include the physical and emotional journey of transformation. She considers the book her love letter to an industry that has provided her professional success but more importantly, a deep connection with people and an outlook that inspires others for positive growth. Whether your looking to be empowered, educated or want an inside look into the world of aesthetics, this author provides you with a must-read.

http://www.mycoachmd.com

CPSIA information can be obtained
at www.ICGtesting.com
Printed in the USA
LVHW011151211219
641338LV00005B/38/P